Also by Klaus Truemper

Brain Science

Artificial Intelligence
Wittgenstein and Brain Science
Magic, Error, and Terror

History

The Daring Invention of Logarithm Tables
The Construction of Mathematics

Technical

Logic-based Intelligent Systems
Effective Logic Computation
Matroid Theory

Edited by Ingrid and Klaus Truemper

F. Hülster *Introduction to Wittgenstein's*
Tractatus Logico-Philosophicus
(English and German edition)

F. Hülster *Berlin 1945: Surviving the Collapse*

SUBCONSCIOUS BLUNDERS

A 21st-CENTURY EPIDEMIC

KLAUS TRUEMPER

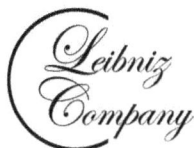

Leibniz Company

Softcover published by Leibniz Company
2304 Cliffside Drive
Plano, Texas, 75023
USA

Original edition 2023
Updated edition 2024

The book is typeset in LATEX using the Tufte-style book class, which was inspired by the work of Edward R. Tufte and Richard Feynman.

Sources and licenses for all figures are listed in the Notes section.

Library of Congress Cataloging-in-Publication Data
Truemper, Klaus, 1942–

Subconscious Blunders: A 21st-Century Epidemic
ISBN 978-0-9991402-7-7
1. Subconscious. 2. Neuroscience. 3. Epidemic.

Contents

1

Introduction

Our nervous system—the brain, the spinal cord, and the network of nerves—delivers an astonishing performance. The *conscious mind*[1] is the top part of that wondrous system. The rest is the *subconscious*. It supplies the input for the conscious mind.

In recent decades, several forces have spurred the subconscious of virtually everyone to produce vast amounts of erroneous input to the conscious. It truly is an epidemic of subconscious errors.

Let's look at some examples.

Examples of Subconscious Errors

- Every day, John spends hours on Facebook and Twitter.[2] When he publishes a post, he feels compelled to check every few minutes whether others have commented favorably.
- Two hours after a meal, John feels hungry and needs to eat again. In response, he fetches a snack.
- During an annual physical exam, the doctor tells John that his cholesterol is way up, as is his blood pressure. The doctor prescribes two pills. John agrees to take them to fix these problems.

The three situations have in common that a feeling or unbidden thought triggers an erroneous decision. Let's see:

- The feeling "I wonder what others think about my post" impels John to check for "likes" every few minutes. He is disappointed when only a few have cared to respond.
Result: He becomes depressed.

- The feeling of hunger two hours after a meal causes him to overeat.
Result: His weight goes up and up.

- The unbidden thought "Good that medication can fix this" triggers John's acceptance of the doctor's recommendation.
Result: The drugs have nasty side effects. John has muscle pain and feels dizzy and weak.

Where do the feelings and unbidden thoughts come from? They certainly aren't the result of deliberate thinking since they just pop up. Well, they come from the subconscious. Their key characteristic is that they show up without any perceivable justification. They simply *happen*. They result in major harm in each of the cited cases.

Are there more situations of this kind? Yes, indeed, we are engulfed in them. Here's why.

Central Role of Subconscious Output

How does the conscious mind obtain any information about the body or the world? There is only one way: The subconscious must produce the information in the form of feelings and unbidden thoughts.

How can this be? Don't we directly see things, hear words, sense heat, touch surfaces, taste food, and so on?

Yes, it does seem that we directly accomplish this, doesn't it? Actually, in each case subconscious processes make the conscious sensation possible.

For example, when photons enter the eyes, subconscious processes convert the information into signals and send them to a portion of the brain where other subconscious processes analyze the information and eventually assemble an image that pops up in consciousness.

As far as the conscious mind is concerned, the image shows up without any deliberate effort. But it actually results from very sophisticated subconscious processing. Technically, we consider the image to be part of the unbidden thoughts that the subconscious outputs to the conscious mind.

Whenever the subconsciously produced feelings and thoughts are flawed, the conscious mind operates on the basis of incorrect information and arrives at wrong or harmful decisions and actions.

How often does the subconscious create erroneous output? Right now, in the 21st century, lots and lots of times.

We focus on two causes: evolution, or rather a lack of appropriate evolution, and actions of our profit-driven economic system.

Evolution

The human race, with all its capabilities and frailties, is the end result of millions of years of evolution. During that vast period, the world changed substantially a number of times. The changes happened at a pace slow enough that evolution could track them, in the sense that organisms either adapted or were replaced. That included the development of the human race, where *Homo sapiens* was the final outcome.

For the last 10,000 years, humans have caused changes at a much more rapid pace. It began when they cleared trees and brush to plant crops, introduced irrigation, and domesticated animals.

The pace gradually increased, and today changes happen with dizzying speed. Humans create something new literally every day: new materials, new medicines, new machines, ... The list seems endless.

On the time scale of evolution, the last 10,000 years are just a blip. As a result, evolution could not keep up and modify the subconscious so that the output of feelings and unbidden thoughts is always appropriate.

Indeed, the subconscious fails to properly function lots of times, resulting in major disasters. For example, due to faulty evolutionary programming, humans conduct wars, gradually destroy land and oceans, deplete natural resources, and eliminate many species of animals. In some sense, humans have become a scourge of the Earth.

Recent decades have added a new dimension to the failures of the subconscious.

Profit Motive

Industry has created products that subtly alter the processes of the subconscious. That manipulation has produced huge profits. But it also has caused, and is still causing, extraordinary harm. For example:

- Social media platforms suggest topics to the user with the goal that the user stays connected as long as possible. This strategy maximizes advertising revenue. It has the insidious side effect that it alters the subconscious. Among the changes, physical violence becomes an acceptable strategy for pursuing one's goals.

  In Myanmar, wild conspiracy theories on Facebook fueled the genocide of the minority Muslim Rohingya.[3] At least 25,000 were killed, tens of thousands raped, and more than 700,000 fled abroad.[4]

- Food and drink designed by the food industry and related advertising have changed subconscious evaluations of when, where, what, and how much one should eat and drink.[5]

  In particular, eating has become an addiction that demands food and drink far beyond physical needs. That change is one of the major causes for the obesity crisis of the US, where 42% of adults were obese in 2022.[6]

- Intensive promotion of opioids for pain treatment by pharmaceutical companies changed subconscious processes. Taking a pill became much more attractive than physical efforts to control pain. The change triggered the opioid crisis in the US. So far more than 100,000 people have died of drug overdoses.[7]

You might say that these disasters, while horrific, are isolated instances that have no connection with your life.

Sorry, that argument is not correct. For example, the strategy of social media that propelled the genocide in Myanmar also has a major negative impact on the subconscious of users in the US, leading to pathological computer use, eating disorders, social anxiety, lowered self-esteem, and even suicide.[8] As another example, the marketing push by the pharmaceutical industry doesn't just involve opioids, but a vast array of other, often unneeded, medicines.

In fact, as we shall see, the cited instances are just the tip of an iceberg of problems that affect virtually everyone. They have in common that subconscious processes produce wrong feelings and unbidden thoughts that, in turn, prod the conscious mind into wrong decisions and actions.

Remedy

"Oh my," you likely think, "will this book lay out disaster after disaster, and then boldly suggest a global cure that restructures the subconscious of billions of people?"

Don't worry, we won't assemble such a global prescription. In fact, we have no idea how it could be formulated and implemented.[9]

But we *can* pursue the following goal. Each of us can make changes so that our subconscious no longer falls prey to these manipulations. We thus can improve important parts of our life.

How do we obtain the required insight? We use brain science for that purpose. It helps us understand how the subconscious creates feelings and unbidden thoughts. With that information, we can analyze the errors of the subconscious, and—more importantly— how we can restructure the subconscious to avoid them.

Surprised? How can we possibly change the subconscious, given that, by definition, we don't have conscious insight into its inner workings? Well, it can be done, as we see in the chapters to come.

Don't worry, this won't be a boring discussion of theoretical claims and proofs. Instead, we will crisscross a terrain of practical problems. Each step increases insight into the role of feelings and unbidden thoughts produced by the subconscious, and how we can change the subconscious to eliminate erroneous output.

Prior Work

A number of books cover shortcomings of human decision making. In particular, intuitive choices produced by the subconscious have proved to be both right and wrong in numerous settings. Three books investigate intuition-based decision making in great detail:

- *Thinking, Fast and Slow*[10] by D. Kahneman
- *The Invisible Gorilla*[11] by C. Chabris and D. Simons
- *Intuition*[12] by D. Myers

Related is the concept of *overthinking*. Numerous texts cover that topic.[13] The book *Stop Overthinking*[14] by N. Trenton deserves particular mention.

These books consider flawed output by the subconscious while conscious thoughts deal with some decision problem. In this book we look at different situations where erroneous feelings and unbidden thoughts simply pop up and cause havoc.

Several books discuss the horrible results when the subconscious is manipulated for profit. Five key references:

- *The Hungry Gene: The Inside Story of the Obesity Crisis*[15] by E. R. Shell

- *Salt Sugar Fat: How the Food Giants Hooked Us*[16] by M. Moss

- *Digital Minimalism: Choosing a Focused Life in a Noisy World*[17] by C. Newport

- *The Chaos Machine: The Inside Story of How Social Media Rewired Our Minds and Our World*[18] by M. Fisher

- *Dopamine Nation: Finding Balance in the Age of Indulgence*[19] by A. Lembke

Use of the Book

Two thoughts:

First, we firmly believe that pleasurable results not earned by serious effort invariably turn out to be fleeting and ultimately vacuous. On the other hand, when we work hard to attain something, the reward will last for a while, in some cases even decades. The book is written in that spirit: It calls for commitment and significant actions, and sometimes for hard work. In turn, the book promises major improvements.

Second, the proposals of this book aren't some ideas that just sounded good to us. We have implemented them for ourselves and obtained major improvements in our life.

But—isn't there always a "But"?—there isn't a universal standard for appropriate living, and some suggestions may be at odds with your philosophy of life. The best we can suggest is that you examine each conclusion of the book, think about its usefulness for your life, and then adopt or ignore ideas as you see fit.

Before we analyze the role of the subconscious in our lives, we need to cover some technical aspects of brain science. The next chapter contains that material. By the way, the technical term for brain science is *neuroscience*. We use it from now to be consistent with the literature.

2

Nervous System

Modern neuroscience started in the 1990s. Since then, neuroscientists have assembled a rich body of theory about the nervous system and its interaction with the rest of the body. Yet, the numerous results still are like isolated pieces of a vast mosaic that, we hope, eventually will supply coherent insight into human reasoning.

How can these partial results help us today to cope with intricate problems of life, such as described in the introduction? Aren't the existing pieces of the theory too disparate to guide us?

The answer: One should design a hypothesis about the overall functioning of the nervous system from the numerous isolated results, then use that hypothesis to investigate human problems of interest.

We developed such a hypothesis in prior work; the books *Wittgenstein and Brain: Understanding the World*[20] and *Artificial Intelligence: Why AI Projects Succeed or Fail*[21] have details. There we investigated two disparate areas: Philosophy, where we studied philosophical problems that had been unsolved for centuries, and Computer Science, where we established some principles for the design and implementation of intelligent machines.

This chapter summarizes the architecture of the nervous system and introduces basic aspects of the hypothesis.

Architecture

The nervous system consists of the *brain*, the *spinal cord*, and the *network of nerves* that connect the brain and the spinal cord to other parts of the human body, for example, to the eyes, ears, organs, muscles, blood vessels, and glands.[22] Here is a drawing showing the components.

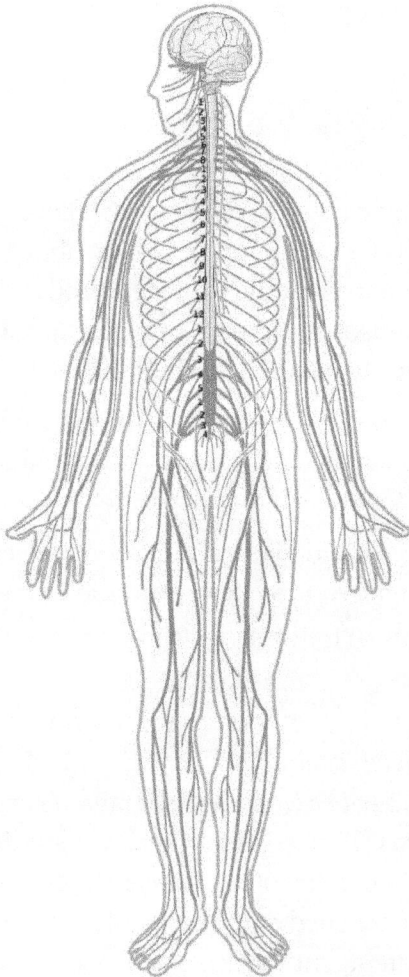

Nervous system diagram.[23]

Neuroprocesses

In principle, the nervous system functions as follows. The network of nerves picks up information coming from outside the body such as signals coming from the eyes and ears, as well as from the body itself such as the level of oxygen in the bloodstream.

Various parts of the nervous system such as the brain and the spinal cord process the incoming data. The resulting insight triggers responses that may occur just inside the body such as a change in the heart rate, or outside such as the driver of a car stepping on the brakes.

It gets more complicated when one tries to trace how information flows exactly, which part of the system does what, and how all of this is controlled.

We define a much simplified version that accommodates all of these operations. To this end, we declare any process in the body that involves information acquisition and subsequent reaction in any form, to be a *neuroprocess*. We use this term knowing full well that some neuroprocesses take place in part or wholly outside the nervous system.

We are aware of some of the neuroprocesses while others escape conscious attention. We call the neuroprocesses we are aware of *conscious*, and the rest *subconscious*. With these two concepts we characterize the complex information flow of the nervous system as follows.

- Information from the outside world or the body into the nervous system: It is the input into the subconscious neuroprocesses. Examples: Photons entering the eyes, temperature sensed by the skin, and the level of sugar in the bloodstream.

- Information flowing from the subconscious neuroprocesses to the conscious ones: It consists of feelings and unbidden thoughts produced by the subconscious neuroprocesses. They pop up in consciousness without any perceivable justification.

Examples: an image of the surroundings, feeling hungry, and the thought "I shouldn't have done that."

- The conscious neuroprocesses accept the feelings und unbidden thoughts of the subconscious processes, engage in deliberate thoughts, and come up with decisions and actions.
Examples: the decisions "I need to put on a coat" and stepping on the brakes.

To summarize: Information from the world and the body is the input for the subconscious neuroprocesses. In turn, they output feelings and unbidden thoughts to the conscious neuroprocesses, which in turn use deliberate thoughts to establish decisions and actions. A diagram summarizes the process. The flow of information starts at the bottom with world and body data, proceeds upward, and ends at the top with decisions and actions.

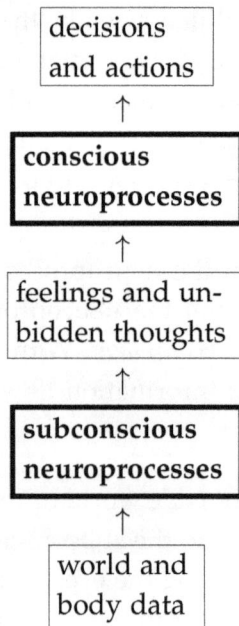

```
┌─────────────────┐
│ decisions       │
│ and actions     │
└─────────────────┘
         ↑
┌─────────────────┐
│ conscious       │
│ neuroprocesses  │
└─────────────────┘
         ↑
┌─────────────────┐
│ feelings and un-│
│ bidden thoughts │
└─────────────────┘
         ↑
┌─────────────────┐
│ subconscious    │
│ neuroprocesses  │
└─────────────────┘
         ↑
┌─────────────────┐
│ world and       │
│ body data       │
└─────────────────┘
```

The diagram seems too simple to be useful, doesn't it? Well, we accommodate lots of situations with that formulation. For example, vision data enter the eyes, subconscious neuroprocesses analyze the information, and the perceived visual impression pops up in consciousness. There, deliberate thoughts come up with a reaction, for example, moving the steering wheel of the car to avoid an obstacle.

Nevertheless, you are right: The diagram *is* simplistic. For example, it doesn't accommodate learning of subconscious neuroprocesses. We introduce these enhancements later as the need arises.

Grouping of Errors

We can group erroneous feelings and unbidden thoughts in several ways. For example, according to:

- The causes that produce them, such as evolution, upbringing, and industry influence.

- An overall theme that one could call *imagined versus actual needs*. Imagined needs prompt the subconscious neuroprocesses to create erroneous feelings and unbidden thoughts that fail to address actual needs.

- A classification according to the parts of life affected by the erroneous feelings and unbidden thoughts.

The first and second ways seem like a dry discussion of science where the root causes are covered one by one. The third view seems more interesting since it shows where and how various errors affect our functioning in life.

In that spirit, we begin with cases where erroneous feelings and unbidden thoughts affect our physical well-being.

Part I

Body

3
Cold and Hot

Let's start with a simple situation.

It's a December morning in Texas. You step outside the house to fetch the newspaper. It's 40 degrees F. Oh boy, it's cold again!

At the same time, in Honolulu it's 67 degrees F, in Florida 50 degrees F, and in Iowa 20 degrees F. No matter. Whoever steps outside to get the newspaper reacts the same way: Oh my, it's cold!

How is such an identical assessment of entirely different temperatures possible?

The answer: Subconscious neuroprocesses perceive the temperature reduction via the skin. They predict that the change will be damaging to the body, based on a hypothesis that the low temperature will persist. Indeed, the subconscious neuroprocesses anticipate hypothermia, illness, even death. No wonder these neuroprocesses issue a feeling of hurt and pain as a warning. The conscious neuroprocesses respond and decide that we must move immediately to a warmer temperature.

Correct Interpretation

The alarm would be well justified if we were planning to stay outside for an extended period and it were truly cold. But in the current case it's plain silly. Grabbing the newspaper and returning to the house takes less than 30 seconds. During that time, even the cold air in Iowa cannot possibly lower the body temperature in any significant way.

A similar situation. It's August. You return from the supermarket to the parking lot and step into the car. It's 100 degrees F inside the car. You react, "Boy, is this hot!" Panicked, you start the engine and turn on the air conditioning.

As soon as cool air exits the vents, you relax and feel better. Yet, with or without air conditioning, the body temperature will not change to any significant extent during the next five minutes. Subconscious neuroprocesses are responsible for the exaggerated reaction. They assume that the elevated temperature will persist for an extended period and harm the body. No wonder the subconscious neuroprocesses issue panicking thoughts.

———————————

In both the cold and hot cases, the subconscious neuroprocesses output feelings and unbidden thoughts that aren't justified by the circumstances. Why is this happening? How can we turn off, so to speak, these erroneous evaluations while retaining the correct response to truly dangerous situations?[24]

We derive the answers in two steps. First, we determine how the subconscious neuroprocesses create feelings and unbidden thoughts.

4

Models

- How do weather forecasters predict tomorrow's weather?
- How do aeronautical engineers evaluate the design of an airplane?
- How do economists establish strategies preventing a recession?

The answers:

- Weather forecasters define and operate mathematical models that accept input about the current weather and then output the forecast.
- Aeronautical engineers build a physical model of the plane and fly it, so to speak, in a wind tunnel.
- Economists create a mathematical model of the economy, input the current situation, introduce various strategies, and compute the effects via the model.

Consider similar questions about the performance of the neuroprocesses:

- How do the neuroprocesses control heart rate, blood pressure, and oxygen intake?
- How do they control the body for appropriate interaction with the world, such as moving the limbs?

- How do they cope with the world in a larger sense, for example, to understand the cause of the tides of the oceans, or why the moon stays in an orbit around the earth?

In short, how do the neuroprocesses control the body's functioning and the interaction with the world? In particular, how do they subconsciously create feelings and unbidden thoughts, and consciously made decisions and actions?

Models Created by Neuroprocesses

The following postulate answers all such questions.[25]

> *The neuroprocesses operate* models *each of which accepts some input and produces relevant output.*

The universality of the postulate is extraordinary. Stephen Hawking calls it *model-dependent realism.*[26]

Here are details for the above situations.

- The subconscious neuroprocesses operate a model that establishes oxygen and carbon dioxide levels in the blood. Based on that information, a model decides the heart rate.

- The subconscious neuroprocesses create models for muscle control of limbs in hundreds of thousands of trials starting in infancy, then rely on these models as demands for action come up.

- The conscious neuroprocesses build models of the world covering the tides of the oceans, the orbits of the moon and the planets, how heat propagates from a stove, and so on. In the distant past, each generation communicated these models to the next one as part of tradition. The advent of writing brought a huge expansion of models since they could be stored.

Direct Actions

You may have noticed that the above discussion includes cases of subconscious operations that go beyond the production of feelings and unbidden thoughts. An example is control of the heart rate. We call such output of the subconscious neuroprocesses *direct actions*.

These actions may be hidden from conscious view, such as control of the heart rate, or they just pop up and can be consciously perceived, for example, when a tap below the knee causes the lower leg to jerk forward.

Enlarged Diagram

We expand the diagram of Chapter 2 to include direct actions of subconscious neuroprocesses. We also add explicit references to the models used by both types of neuroprocesses.

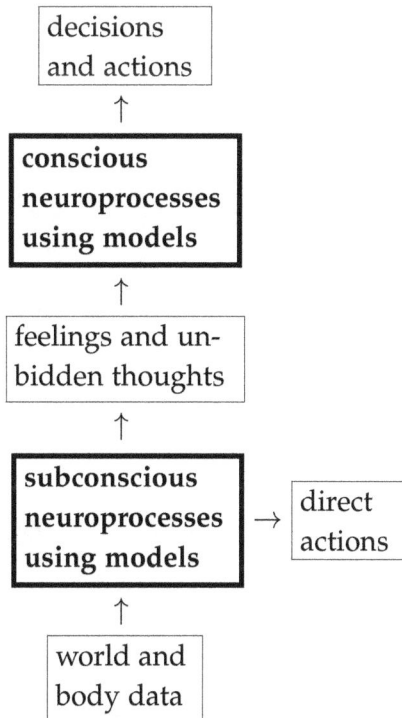

```
          decisions
          and actions
              ↑
        conscious
        neuroprocesses
        using models
              ↑
        feelings and un-
        bidden thoughts
              ↑
        subconscious        direct
        neuroprocesses  →   actions
        using models
              ↑
          world and
          body data
```

Where do the models come from? The next chapter provides the answer.

5
Creation of Models

Where do all those subconscious and conscious models come from? More precisely, who or what creates them?

Evolution has designed the nervous system so that it has some models built in, so to speak. For example, they cope with fundamental control of the body, such as the heartbeat, respiratory rate, and body temperature.

More importantly, evolution has produced the capacity of the nervous system to derive or absorb models. In particular, a baby, child, or adult may acquire a model by trial and error, but also may create it based on direct insight or instruction.

We may view the entire educational process as a huge model-building operation. Indeed, we change models constantly by reading newspapers, interacting with others, carrying out work, and so on. It is a wondrous multifaceted process.

Model Errors

At times, conscious or subconscious models are wrong and cause havoc.[27]

When conscious models fail, we are aware of the error and can consciously work out an improved model. The sciences do so every day when research uncovers new insights and replaces old models with new ones.

The situation is more complicated when models of the sub-conscious fail. By definition, we have no direct understanding of those models and experience only the output of feelings, unbidden thoughts, and direct actions.

When that output is flawed, there may be no warning that it is incorrect. Indeed, we may accept it and derive erroneous decisions and actions.

Panic attacks are an example. Say, we suddenly have the frightening feeling that our heart is failing and we are dying. The heart pounds, we break out in a cold sweat and feel so weak that we lie down. Yet, this is just theater by the body: There is no heart attack, as the doctor determines at the hospital.

With suitable psychotherapy we can learn how to identify panic attacks and react appropriately. From then on, we no longer take a panic attack at face value, but realize that it is a faked disaster.

The example illustrates an important aspect of subconscious errors. We may be totally ignorant that a subconscious model produces erroneous output. Or we are able to analyze that output and see that the subconscious is making a mistake.

The stories about subconscious errors in later chapters reflect these two cases. Sometimes we are not aware that the subconscious has produced an error. At other times we recognize that a mistake has occurred and are able to identify the underlying faulty model of the subconscious.

In either case, we call the mistake a *subconscious error* or, when we want to emphasize the role of models, a *subconscious model error*.

———————

When we become aware of a subconscious model error, we often can employ a certain process and change the flawed model. The next chapter describes how we can accomplish this feat.

6

Remedy

Let's go back to the situation depicted at the beginning of Chapter 3: On a December morning in Texas, you step outside the house to fetch the newspaper. It's 40 degrees. You feel discomfort and shiver. My, is it cold again!

This goes on for several cold mornings, until at some point you wonder: Why do you feel pain when you are outside for half a minute? Surely the cold air cannot cool down your body during that time to any measurable extent.

You think, "This is ridiculous. There is no reason to feel pain."

The process repeats for several days. You walk out, feel pain, and every time think that the pain is not justified. Indeed, the body isn't affected at all by the cold air on that short trip outside.

Effect of Conscious Thoughts

Lo and behold, after several such days the pain lessens and then doesn't set in at all. Instead, as you step outside, your mind wanders, you look toward the horizon, see the first glow of the rising sun, and think, "What a nice day this is!"

What caused the change from pain to the comforting feeling about the start of the day?

The short answer is: The daily repetition of the conscious thought "My body is not affected by the cold air on the short trip outside" gradually changes the model of subconscious neuroprocesses that produces pain when the body senses cold air during the short trip outside.

The claim seems incredible, doesn't it? But it is correct, as we see in a moment.

Mind you, the subconscious neuroprocesses still produce pain when you walk for an extended period in cold air and the body temperature drops. But for the specific case of the morning excursion, the above thought refines the model producing such pain, and the morning excursion creates a different response.

Main Claim

The above case of a conscious thought changing a model of subconscious neuroprocesses isn't an isolated instance. Here is the general claim:

> *Deliberate thoughts of conscious neuroprocesses can change models of subconscious neuroprocesses and thus alter their output of feelings and unbidden thoughts.*

The claim has been proved time and again by cognitive behavioral therapy (CBT). Let's look at that approach of psychotherapy.

Cognitive Behavioral Therapy (CBT)

In traditional approaches to psychotherapy, the therapist helps the patient understand the problem. The patient then acts upon that insight.

Cognitive behavioral therapy (CBT) is different. It is based on the postulate that thought distortions result in destructive feelings and behavior. Hence, the therapist helps the patient to think differently, with the effect that the patient abandons the negative feelings and behavior.

The key statement is:

> *Our deliberate thoughts trigger our feelings, therefore changing our thoughts will change our feelings.*[28]

CBT has proved to be effective for a variety of disorders, for example, for depression, anxiety, alcohol and drug abuse, and eating disorders.[29]

When we rephrase the key statement of CBT using subconscious and conscious neuroprocesses and the related models, we get the earlier claim:

> *Deliberate thoughts of conscious neuroprocesses can change models of subconscious neuroprocesses and thus alter their output of feelings and unbidden thoughts.*

Changing Direct Action

Up to this point we have considered changes of subconscious models that produce feelings and unbidden thoughts. But the same conclusion applies to direct actions taken by subconscious neuroprocesses. That is, conscious thoughts can influence the subconscious production of direct actions.

For example, conscious thoughts during meditation—in particular mindfulness—gradually change the model controlling heart rate.[30]

Enlarged Diagram

We expand the diagram of Chapter 4 so that it includes the effect of consciously produced, deliberate thoughts on subconscious models.

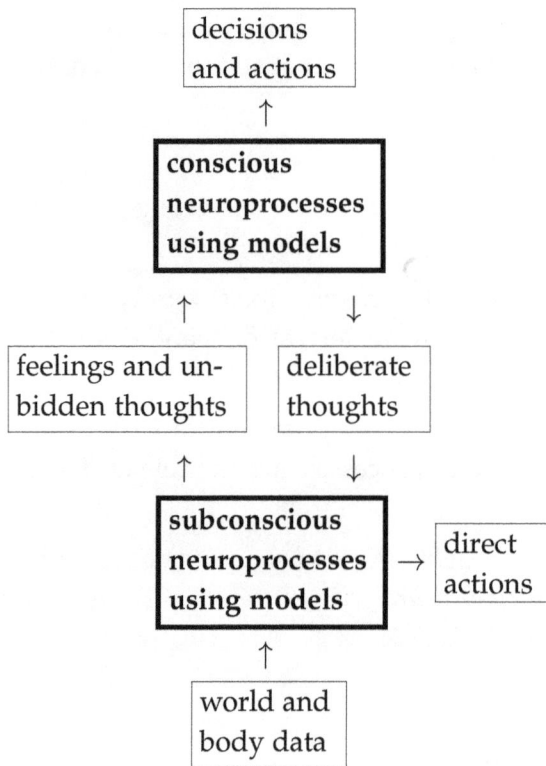

```
        ┌──────────────┐
        │ decisions    │
        │ and actions  │
        └──────────────┘
               ↑
   ┌────────────────────┐
   │ conscious          │
   │ neuroprocesses     │
   │ using models       │
   └────────────────────┘
        ↑              ↓
┌──────────────┐  ┌──────────────┐
│ feelings and un-│ │ deliberate   │
│ bidden thoughts │ │ thoughts     │
└──────────────┘  └──────────────┘
        ↑              ↓
   ┌────────────────────┐
   │ subconscious       │      ┌──────────┐
   │ neuroprocesses     │  →   │ direct   │
   │ using models       │      │ actions  │
   └────────────────────┘      └──────────┘
               ↑
        ┌──────────────┐
        │ world and    │
        │ body data    │
        └──────────────┘
```

Two Rivers

You might have the impression that the flow of deliberate thoughts into subconscious neuroprocesses is an occasional event. Far from it. Indeed, it's best to imagine a constant flow of these thoughts, together with the reverse flow of feelings and unbidden thoughts. The appropriate image is of two rivers that continuously flow in opposite directions.

Correction of Negative Feelings and Thoughts

You might say that all this is somewhat interesting, but why should you care that you feel cold while fetching the newspaper?

Actually, negative feelings and unbidden thoughts may pop up throughout the day that upon closer examination aren't justified. In each of these cases, we pause for a moment, examine the situation, and conclude that the subconsciously produced negative feelings and thoughts are wrong.

For example:

- We miss the bus. The negative thought "Made another mistake" flashes up. Analysis brings up the correction "It doesn't really matter, we have plenty of time to get home."

- A swimmer uses our favorite shower at the pool. We have to select another shower that puts out less and only lukewarm water. Whereupon the thought rises, "How annoying, why does this always happen to me?" Reflecting about it for a moment, we tell ourselves, "When I am camping in the mountains, that supposedly inferior shower would be a godsend."

- We sit cramped in an airliner, with a rather large man next to us. The thought "Flying these days is a royal pain" comes up. Pausing for a moment, we counter with, "Think about the maritime explorers of the past who spent weeks or even months under awful conditions to get anywhere." Then sitting a bit crowded during a two-hour flight no longer produces mental anguish.

- We unfold the newspaper and see on the front page the photo of a politician we despise. We feel bad at that moment and think, "Here is another awful situation." Yet there is nothing we can do about it. We argue against the negative reaction by the thought "There is nothing I can do about this criminal." Then we make the even better decision "We shouldn't even look at this stuff."

We reinforce this during vacation by imposing a *news fast*: We do not read newspapers, watch TV, or surf the Internet for news. When we get back into our routine, we realize how much of that daily flood of information is useless drivel that clutters our mind.

Convinced, we decide to ignore that useless information from now on. Sitting in an airport terminal with TVs blaring political news, we move to a quiet corner and read a book.

In each case, the new thoughts yield an immediate improvement: The response overrides the negative feeling. When the situation recurs, the deliberate corrective thoughts gradually change the underlying subconscious models. When we do this consistently, the negative feelings and unbidden thoughts subside and are replaced by comforting ones. The result is a more relaxed and happier life.

Psychotherapists sometimes hand out the advice "Don't sweat the small stuff." After a short pause, they continue, "It's all small stuff."[31] We would add, "Eliminate the small stuff with positive thoughts."

———————————

In the remainder of this part we look at other erroneous feelings and unbidden thoughts that concern our body. Next is an all-important case.

7

Food and Drink

The air, with its life-sustaining oxygen, is the most important ingredient for human life. Next in importance are food and drink since they supply energy and replenish fluids. Accordingly, evolution has created sophisticated ways to choose and process food and drink.

Various components of the nervous system carry out these tasks. Receptors of the mouth[32] decide whether food or drink is useful or not. The sophisticated evaluation involves not only the taste, but also the texture, such as crunchiness or gooeyness.

Enteric Nervous System (ENS)

If food passes the test, the enteric nervous system (ENS) takes over control. The system looks deceptively simple: Two thin layers of some 500 million neurons line the esophagus, the stomach, and the small and large intestines.[33]

The ENS decides when food is needed or, conversely, when that need has been satisfied. It stimulates the muscles of the digestive system that propel the food. It meters chemicals that are secreted into the digestive process. It controls the extraction of nutrients, and finally regulates the discharge of unusable material.

The ENS communicates with the brain electrically and chemically: electrically via the vagus nerve and prevertebral ganglia, and chemically via the secretion of neurotransmitters such as acetylcholine, dopamine, and serotonin into the bloodstream. It's no wonder that the ENS is often called "the second brain."[34]

Part of the communication of the ENS and the mouth receptors with the brain consists of feelings and unbidden thoughts at the consciousness level. They convey whether food or drink is good for us or bad, whether we should acquire more food or drink or, conversely, stop the intake. The feelings may even include happiness.

Evolution created all this over eons. In particular, evolution arranged it that certain foods and drinks taste particularly good to guarantee consumption.

The food processing industry has tampered with these natural preferences to maximize profits, as we see next.

8

Sugar, Fat, and Salt

Cells in the human body generate energy by combining oxygen with sugar. The bloodstream supplies these ingredients and removes the resulting carbon dioxide (CO_2) and water.

Going backward in the sequence of events, the digestive processes described in Chapter 7 derive the sugar from food and drink and place it into the bloodstream. The respiratory system supplies the oxygen.

Reaction to Sugar, Fat, and Salt

Pure sugar doesn't occur in nature except for rare instances, such as the honey collected by bees. Hence evolution was forced to create a complex digestive system that derives sugar from other carbohydrates, proteins, and fat.

- When sugar or sugar substitutes such as high-fructose corn syrup[35] are added to food and drink and thus directly tossed into the digestive machinery, it's like pouring gasoline onto a smoldering fire: The receptors in the mouth trigger a rush of pleasant feelings, even happiness.

- Fat can be stored in the body and is essential to sustain life during lean times. Due to this importance, food containing fat produces strong positive feelings just like sugar.

- Salt and certain other minerals are essential for the sophisticated life-sustaining processes of the human body. Since nature doesn't supply them readily, the digestive system has been designed to extract them from food and drink. As with sugar and fat, these minerals generate a flood of pleasant reactions. In particular, the addition of salt to food almost magically improves taste.

Food Manipulation

Suppose you want to create foods and drinks that are irresistible to shoppers. How would you do this? Well, it's easy to achieve: You add sugar, fat, and salt to existing food or, more boldly, to some combination of food components. In the latter case, you focus on cheap components. Eaten by themselves, these components might taste bland, even awful. But with the addition of sugar, fat, and salt, they suddenly taste wonderful.

Optimization

To optimize the selection process, you assemble various versions of a given food or drink, test them for taste, and use the results to build a mathematical model that predicts taste based on the ingredients and added sugar, fat, and salt.

You apply a sophisticated computer program to the model. It computes a formula where the food or drink not only tastes best, but among the ways to achieve that result, can be produced at minimum cost.

This simple description of optimized food construction suffices for our purposes. In reality, the design of optimized food and drink is more complicated. For example, sugar helps improve taste only up to a certain point, and it interacts with fat in the production of taste in a complicated way. The book *Salt Sugar Fat: How the Food Giants Hooked Us*[36] by M. Moss covers the history of these developments and key facts, including the extraordinary marketing effort to convince the public that the consumption of these foods is essential for a happy life.

It seems reasonable that we declare any food or drink created by the above process to be *optimized*. That definition stays clear of any controversy surrounding the classification of food and drink as unprocessed, minimally processed, processed, and ultra-processed based on ingredients and manufacturing methods.[37] Optimized foods and drinks include all ultra-processed cases as well as some processed ones.

Harmful Effects

When a pharmaceutical company proposes treatment of some disease with a novel drug, they must establish two results before they can market the product: They must show that the treatment is effective, and that it doesn't have harmful side effects.

No such standard exists for optimized food. Companies can create new products and market them, with no official approval needed. Admittedly, showing that an optimized food is safe and doesn't produce harmful effects isn't easy since the damage may show up only after years of consumption.

But wouldn't you expect that, once those years have passed, any product that in hindsight can be demonstrated to be harmful, must be discontinued or at least reformulated?

But that's not happening. We now know that many optimized foods and drinks are grossly harmful, yet no law calls for bans or reformulation. The next chapter has the dismal details.

9

A Health Crisis

At all times of recorded history, some people overindulged in food and drink and became overweight or even obese.[38] Recent decades have seen something very different: an ever growing epidemic of obesity. For example, the obesity rate in the US more than tripled from 13% of adults in 1960 to 42% in 2022.[39]

What has changed in people's lives to cause such a dramatic increase? One factor stands out: The rise of optimized foods and drinks to the point where it's almost impossible to avoid them. According to one study, optimized food and drink contributed in 2019 more than 60% of the energy of diets in the US.[40]

As we have seen, optimized food and drink have been designed to create a very pleasing eating and drinking experience. They even produce happiness. But they also reduce the effectiveness of signals by the enteric nervous system (ENS) to stop eating. The result: The body gains a little more weight every day, with no end in sight.

Obesity

Obesity causes horrific health problems: diabetes, cardiovascular diseases, certain types of cancer, osteoarthritis, anxiety, depression, even cognitive decline.[41]

Politicians seemingly are unable to control this monstrous development via suitable laws. How can we avoid that train wreck for ourselves?

Buying Food and Drink

Say, we walk into a large supermarket. At the entrance are pies and pastries on several tables, racks with rich gourmet cheeses, a deli brimming with dozens of wonderful sausages, hams, and other cured meat. It's a veritable cornucopia of temptation.

As we enter, we engage in a dialogue with ourselves, "Wow, they keep on tempting me, don't they? But I know that this stuff isn't good for me, so let's move on to the vegetable and fruit section."

At first we have to initiate that dialogue with conscious thought. But after a few weeks, it becomes automatic: Models in our subconscious neuroprocesses have changed as predicted by cognitive behavioral therapy (CBT), and we react differently.

As we enter the supermarket, a subconsciously produced message comes up, "Yeah, this stuff looks good but is really bad for me." In fact, we develop an aversion against these products. The more negative the thought, the better for us.

Decisions, Decisions

When you consider canned food or baked goods, first scan the label for salt, sugar, and fat content, and reject the food outright when the quantities are excessive.

Next, check the list of ingredients. At times you will be shocked by the large variety of added chemicals. Be aware that manufacturers may disguise ingredients.

For example, the label of a cereal package may list "Malted barley." You think, "Oh, the barley has been processed a bit." No, it means that the barley has been coated with sugar. This fact cannot be disguised on the list of contents. There it is: Sugar is listed as 5 gram per serving of 58 gram. That's not so bad for a cereal, considering that sugar content of optimized cereal ranges up to 50%.

Not buying foods that are bad for us is only part of the cure. In the US it's the norm that most every adult who hasn't retired yet has a full-time job. Preparing meals at home seems too much to ask, so we go out and eat in fast-food places.

Fast Food

The fast-food industry has changed dramatically. Here is an example. When we ordered a hamburger from McDonald's in the 1960s, we got a bun with a slim slice of grilled hamburger meat and a bit of mayonnaise and mustard.

That hamburger is the emaciated cousin of current hamburgers. They have one or two hefty slices of grilled hamburger meat and thick slices of cheese and bacon. Just one of these monsters supplies almost one fourth of the total calories needed for the day.

It's even worse if we order soda pop as a beverage since it is loaded with sugar or other sweeteners. We compound the error if we substitute a large milk shake for the soda pop. The hamburger and shake together supply half of the total calories for the day.

What can we do about this? Plainly speaking, we simply don't go to fast food places except, maybe, to have one of their salads with a drink of water.

How will we have the strength to drive past those places? Every time we see one, we tell ourselves, "That food is not good for me." After a while it becomes an automatic response by subconscious neuroprocesses. It's a mantra for survival.

More on Decisions

We are not done yet. Since we are now cooking almost every meal at home, we need to learn to make the right decisions in the super-market.

We buy fruits and vegetables; small amounts of fish and chicken, almost no red meat; low- or non-fat milk; non-fat yogurt; some cheeses that aren't overly rich in fat; some eggs, rice, and regular or sweet potatoes. Definitely no soda pop or other artificially sweetened drinks.

We prepare the foods in a variety of ways using little oil and salt, maybe even adopt an entire cuisine such as Chinese cooking. Since bread offered in the supermarket usually contains lots of salt, we bake whole-grain bread using minimal amounts of salt. Indeed, the ingredients should just be water, flour, grain, and a small amount of salt. We make the bread rise using sourdough—our preference— or yeast.[42]

Conscious thoughts have produced the revised models that our subconscious neuroprocesses now operate for food selection. We praise ourselves each time we make a good decision, and argue against bad choices.

After a while, the new models of the subconscious neuroprocesses automatically reproduce those comments in their output. At that point we have won the battle.

Counter Arguments

Sounds too easy, doesn't it? Yes, you are right. The change is difficult. At first, the food you prepare tastes bland. No wonder, it's missing all that sugar, fat, and salt. Drinking water instead of sweet soda seems dull.

Then slowly but surely your tastebuds adapt—that is, their models change—and you notice a reverse effect: Whenever you sample optimized food, it tastes overly sweet, too rich in fat, and too salty. When you sample soda pop, the sickly sweet taste is revolting.

Food now tastes pleasant but doesn't supply the rush engineered into optimized food. Most importantly, the message "We have eaten enough and should stop" sent by the enteric nervous system (ENS) to the brain results in the desired action.

In the end you discover a new freedom: You have overcome the addiction and once more control what enters your body. What a wonderful feeling!

"Yes," you might agree, "all this sounds wonderful, except that I don't have time for all this food preparation." Indeed, something else needs to be given up. How about reducing activities on social media, another modern affliction that we look at later?

Mantras help here, too. For example, telling yourself time and again, "This food will really be great for me; I cannot wait to sit down and enjoy it." It gradually builds an enjoyment of food preparation, just as CBT predicts.

Yes, It's Like Alcoholism

Somebody might say, "No, you really don't have to do all that. Simply consume less of the wonderful industry-produced foods and drinks. That way you get the terrific eating experience, yet don't gain weight."

The argument overlooks that the optimized foods and drinks are so designed that the enteric nervous system (ENS) no longer sends a timely and effective signal to stop eating.

Hence the advice "Eat less" is the analog of advising an alcoholic to drink less. It doesn't work.

Specific Plans

The Mediterranean diet[43] and the DASH diet[44] contain detailed instructions for selecting and preparing healthy foods. A newer development, the MIND diet,[45] improves on both diets. It not only assures wonderful nutrition, but helps stem cognitive decline and lowers the incidence of Alzheimer's disease.

The book *How Not to Die: Discover the Foods Scientifically Proven to Prevent and Reverse Disease*[46] discusses in great detail how certain foods are harmful and cause or contribute to diseases, while others promote health.

A Deceptive Claim

When author M. Moss of *Salt Sugar Fat*[47] carried out his research about the horrendous effect of optimized foods, some companies tried to convince him that the addition of salt, sugar, and fat was essential for tasty foods. They demonstrated this by preparing their bread, cookies, and so on without adding any salt, sugar, or fat. Moss confirmed that the food tasted awful. Some of the food looked sickly or felt squishy like mud.

Does this prove that the addition of salt, sugar, and fat cannot be avoided if looks and taste are to be even reasonable? No, it doesn't. The argument overlooks how that food came to be. The optimization process not only evaluates the impact of salt, sugar, and fat, but also how good taste can be achieved with cheapest ingredients. Take bread, for example. As Moss describes, the bread without salt, sugar, and fat looked sickly and tasted awful. But he wasn't told about the ingredients of that awful bread.

As a counterexample, below are two photos of a sourdough bread made of rye flour and hard-wheat flour. For the dough, we add three ingredients: water that is filtered to eliminate chlorine, a sourdough starter, and a tiny amount of salt. We replenish the starter for the next baking using rye flour. The amount of salt is so small that the bread earns the low-sodium classification according to the Food Labeling Guide of the US Food and Drug Administration (FDA).

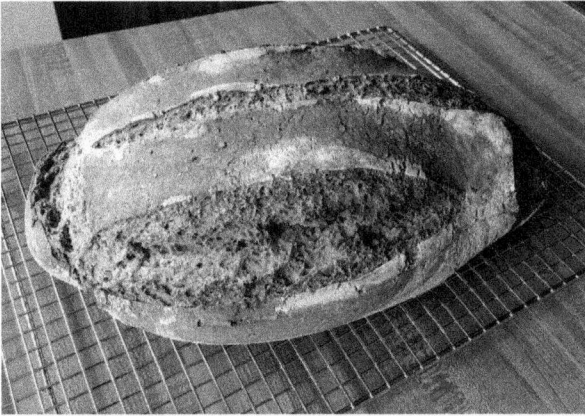

Rye-wheat bread.

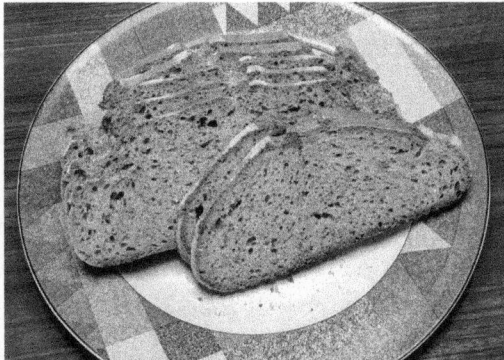

Slices of rye-wheat bread.[48]

The bread tastes wonderful.

Remember the statement that the cells of the body combine sugar with oxygen to create energy? It so happens that subconscious neuroprocesses sometimes propel us to mishandle the acquisition of that oxygen.

Surprised? The next chapter describes how this can happen.

10

Breathless

Chronic obstructive pulmonary disease (COPD) is characterized by breathing problems and poor airflow.[49] The most common symptoms are shortness of breath and a cough that produces sputum.

The disease progresses over time. At present there is no known cure, but the symptoms can be treated and the progression delayed. COPD typically is the result of long-term smoking.

As we shall see, the models of subconscious neuroprocesses guiding breathing deal with COPD rather badly. But one can change the models so that the effects of COPD are much reduced.

The proposed change isn't important just for people afflicted with COPD. To the contrary, everyone can benefit from that change since it generally results in more effective and relaxed breathing.

Let's first look at COPD.

A COPD Case

Robert—not his real name—has COPD. When he exerts any physical effort, he almost immediately feels the need to breathe faster. But regardless how fast he breathes in and out—to the point where he is panting—he still feels that he is not getting enough air. At the same time, his pulse rises significantly.

There is a simple explanation for all this.[50]

The air rushing into Robert's lungs has the life-sustaining oxygen needed by the body. That oxygen is absorbed inside the lungs into the bloodstream. It then travels to all parts of the body, where it is taken up by cells and used to burn carbohydrates. The cells expel the resulting carbon dioxide (CO_2) into the blood, which transports it to the lungs. There, CO_2 becomes part of the air to be exhaled.

For this process to work, the lungs must efficiently absorb oxygen from the inhaled air and place it into the bloodstream. With matching efficiency the lungs must pass CO_2 from the bloodstream into the air to be exhaled.

Due to COPD, Robert's lungs have a significantly reduced capacity for these two functions, and he needs to breathe faster.

Role of Neuroprocesses

In terms of neuroprocesses, we may characterize the situation as follows.

Subconscious neuroprocesses in the *medulla* of the brain operate a suitable model that evaluates the oxygen content in the body's cells.[51]

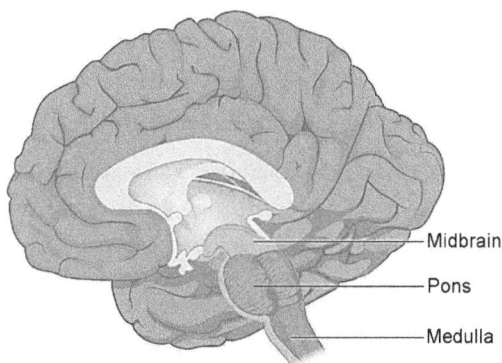

Location of medulla in the brain.[52]

When the oxygen content declines for whatever reason, the model detects this shortcoming, and the subconscious neuroprocesses decide that more rapid breathing and increased blood flow are needed.

Robert normally breathes through the nose. But based on the detected shortcoming, the subconscious neuroprocesses decide that breathing should now be done through the mouth to reduce resistance encountered by the increased volume of air. So without Robert noticing, the breathing switches from nose to mouth.

If the increased breathing and pulse don't have the desired effect, that is, if the oxygen level in the body's cells doesn't go up, the model detects that fact, and the subconscious neuroprocesses output a feeling of breathlessness and ultimately of suffocation to the conscious neuroprocesses.

As that feeling intensifies, Robert's conscious neuroprocesses decide to reduce physical efforts.

Alternately, Robert may increase oxygen content in the inhaled air with supplemental oxygen.

So the output of the subconscious neuroprocesses leaves Robert with two options: Do less, or use supplemental oxygen.

Major Blunder

The decisions made by the subconscious neuroprocesses, and the two resulting conscious options, seem entirely appropriate. But the subconscious neuroprocesses actually commit a major blunder.

The error is the subconscious decision to switch from nose breathing to mouth breathing. That change is supposed to decrease resistance encountered by the increased air flow. It does so, of course.

But the switch also creates a major problem, as we see next.[53]

Imagine oxygen-rich blood flowing past a cell. The cell absorbs some of the oxygen. Once inside the cell, the oxygen reacts with carbohydrates and creates CO_2. Finally, the cell expels the CO_2 into the blood.

The oxygen in the bloodstream is bound by a chemical bond that must be broken if the oxygen is to enter the cell. How is this accomplished?

For the explanation we must replace the simplistic notion that blood leaving the lungs carries only oxygen, while blood going back to the lungs has only CO_2, with the following, more accurate statement:

Blood always contains a mixture of oxygen and CO_2. It's just that the ratio varies: Oxygen-rich blood leaves the lungs, and CO_2-rich blood returns.

It turns out that the ease with which the cell extracts oxygen from the blood depends crucially on the amount of CO_2 in the blood. That is, the more CO_2 is present, the more easily the cell accomplishes this feat.[54]

Thus, efficient extraction of oxygen from the blood doesn't just require plenty of oxygen in the bloodstream, but also a sufficient amount of CO_2.

How can these two goals be achieved?

Well, the oxygen content depends on the amount of oxygen supplied by the lungs.

What about sufficient CO_2 content? Put differently: What action *reduces* CO_2 content in the blood and slows down the transfer of oxygen into the cells?

The answer to the last question is: Rapid breathing depletes CO_2 of the blood.[55]

Downward Spiral

We now have the following out-of-control situation:

When the oxygen level in the cells drops due to physical activity, subconscious neuroprocesses cause a switch to rapid mouth breathing. Then the CO_2 level in the blood drops, and the cells absorb less oxygen.

In response, the subconscious neuroprocesses cause an acceleration of the breathing rate, which further lowers the CO_2 level in the blood, which in turn reduces the oxygen level in the cells even more, and so on.

Eventually, the oxygen level of the cells spirals down to the point where Robert feels he is suffocating.

For recovery, he stops all physical efforts and waits for the breathing to slow down.

Correct Explanation

We just have seen that mouth breathing is wrong. But on the surface, the much slower nose breathing doesn't seem to be an appropriate alternative, since it doesn't push enough oxygen-carrying air into the lungs.

That argument relies on the simplistic notion that the lungs extract *all* oxygen from the inhaled air and replace it by CO_2 to be exhaled.

In reality, the lungs extract only about a quarter of the available oxygen. The rest is exhaled again.[56]

As a result, the slower nose breathing extracts just a bit less oxygen from the air than the more rapid mouth breathing. But the increased CO_2 content of the blood more than makes up for that small oxygen reduction, and results in increased absorption of oxygen by the cells.

Correct Response

The conclusion is: Robert must breathe through the nose even though feelings produced by subconscious neuroprocesses pressure him to switch to mouth breathing.

He can enforce nose breathing through conscious thoughts that override that urge.

A better approach is to systematically change the behavior of the subconscious neuroprocesses so that he automatically breathes appropriately. For this, Robert focuses on proactive thoughts such as "Mouth breathing makes things worse" and "Nose breathing will help."

He also thinks about details of the oxygen-to-CO_2 exchange and uses a watch to determine how long each inhaled and exhaled breath takes. Finally, he observes how the urge for faster breathing subsides as CO_2 content in the blood increases.

Evidently this is another case of the cognitive behavioral therapy (CBT) of Chapter 6.

Robert engages in these thoughts as he carries out his activities, all the time monitoring that his mouth stays closed and breathing is done solely through the nose.

After a few days of this conscious effort the urge to mouth breathe subsides, and slow nose breathing becomes the subconscious choice whether he is at rest or engaged in physical activities.

This also extends to sleeping. The evidence is that, when he awakens during the night, his mouth has not become dry as happened before.

He has solved the problem!

Results

Here are some statistics brought about by the change to nose breathing. Robert is in his 70s. He has smoked for five decades.

- Physical exercise 1: Daily walking.
  - With rapid mouth breathing:
    Walking 3/8 mile is strenuous. Speed not recorded. Pulse is 94 beats per minute (bpm). Oxygen saturation is 94 percent.

- With slower nose breathing:
  On the first day, distance is doubled from 3/8 mile to 3/4 mile, walking at 4 mph. Oxygen saturation climbs from 94 percent to 97 percent. Previous pulse of 94 bpm goes down every day and reaches plateau of 84 bpm within two weeks. After six weeks, distance is increased to 1 mile.

- Physical exercise 2: Walking 50 feet from the house to the mailbox, with a steep elevation drop of six feet. This sounds like a simple task, but isn't easy since he climbs a 12 percent slope back up to the house.

  - With rapid mouth breathing:
    Robert hyperventilates and becomes exhausted, with pulse rate 90-100 bpm.
  - With slower nose breathing:
    The time for inhaling and exhaling is the same as at rest, the pulse stays at 80, the oxygen level has increased, and he no longer feels pressured or exhausted.

Do you recognize something else in the statistics for the second item? There is no way that the short trip to the mailbox should cause Robert to hyperventilate and become exhausted. It surely looks like a mild panic attack.

As a remedy, Robert adds in conscious thoughts of CBT to conquer the panic attack.[57] The improvements are then due to both the nose breathing and the successful fight against the panic attack.

Benefits for Everyone

You may think, "This is interesting, but I don't have COPD and don't see how all this is relevant for me."

To the contrary, nose breathing benefits everyone in many ways. For hundreds of years, nose breathing has been known to be powerful medicine. Since it affects the balance of oxygen and carbon dioxide in the bloodstream, many modern maladies—asthma, anxiety, attention deficit hyperactivity disorder, psoriasis, and more—can be reduced or even reversed. The book *Breath: The New Science of a Lost Art*[58] describes the wonderful effects in great detail.

That book caused us to switch to nose breathing, with results as predicted. For example, breathing rate is slowed, as is heartbeat. Blood pressure is reduced.

How can we achieve consistent nose breathing when for years or even decades we have relied on mouth breathing? We must change the models of the subconscious neuroprocesses that switch us to mouth breathing whenever we inhale without conscious control.

Cognitive behavioral therapy (CBT) advises how we can achieve the change. Whenever we catch ourselves mouth breathing, we engage in intense thoughts such as "Hey, we need to switch to nose breathing, it really is good for us, let's focus on doing it."

After a while, the mantra changes the model of the controlling subconscious neuroprocesses, and nose breathing happens automatically. At that time, the following happens. Whenever we become aware of the newly acquired nose breathing, we smile and think, "I accomplished this. It's great, isn't it?"

Fatigue is another area where subconscious neuroprocesses can mislead us. Let's see why, and how we can process fatigue properly.

11

Fatigue

We are hiking in the mountains: We climb up slopes and descend into valleys, all the time enjoying the scenery. After four hours, we feel tired and decide to rest.[59]

Where does this feeling come from?

First Explanation

An obvious explanation is: The leg muscles determine that they have been stressed and are tired. They send corresponding information to the brain, which translates it to a feeling of fatigue.

Suppose that vague explanation is correct, and a person's statement such as "My legs are getting tired" captures the essence of the situation.

How then is the following possible?

In 1986, Georges Holtyzer of Belgium walked 418 miles in six and a half days. He was not permitted any stops for rest and moved almost 99 percent of the time.[60]

Why do we get a feeling of fatigue after four hours of hiking when Holtyzer could walk more than six days without rest?

Second Explanation

Research into the causes of fatigue started in the 19th century. It led to the explanation that lack of oxygen and buildup of lactate caused muscle fatigue.

Exercise textbooks from the 1930s to today advance this theory.[61] Here are some problems with that claim:[62]

- Even at peak exertion, only about two-thirds of available muscle fibers are active.

- The feeling of fatigue is delayed when music is played during the activity—as is invariably done at exercise clubs.

- When a wall clock is slowed down, people become tired later.

So, something else must be happening.

Emotion

The crucial insight came during the 2010s, when fatigue was recognized as an emotion:[63] The feeling of fatigue is produced by a subconscious neuroprocess to ensure that ongoing physical efforts don't overtax the body.

This insight supports the following explanation of fatigue:

- A subconscious neuroprocess analyzes the performance of the physical body and decides whether the current effort if continued not just for hours but days would cause damage. We aren't consciously aware of this analysis.

- Once the subconscious neuroprocess arrives at that conclusion, it outputs a feeling of fatigue. We recognize that feeling and decide to rest. We can restate this as: A conscious neuroprocess becomes aware of the feeling and concludes that rest is needed.

Thus, fatigue is an emotion that protects the body from harm.

Appropriate Reaction

How, then, should we respond when the fatigue feeling surfaces?

An obvious decision: We rest for a while to give ourselves a breather from the rapid pace of modern life. We can contemplate where we are, what we are doing, and where we are going. We may engage in some meditation and thus slow down the pace. After a few minutes or even half an hour, we rise refreshed to tackle the problems of life again.

There are some situations where the overly cautious output of fatigue interferes with important goals. Let's look at two examples.

Sports

Athletes competing in long-distance races replace unjustified feelings of fatigue with proactive thoughts that gradually replace the models used by subconscious neuroprocesses with different models proposing perseverance. It works, just as cognitive behavioral therapy (CBT) predicts.

The famous Finnish distance runner Paavo Nurmi put it thus:[64]

> "Mind is everything. Muscles are pieces of rubber. All that I am, I am because of my mind."

The new thoughts of perseverance propel the runner until the body reaches its physical limit. This happens in one of two ways:[65]

- The runner has calibrated the effort so carefully that she is at the point of physical exhaustion just as she reaches the finish line. At that moment, perseverance is overtaken by fatigue, and the runner collapses. But minutes later, she is up again and celebrating.

- If the runner has miscalculated and exhaustion sets in before the end of the race, that calamity manifests itself in the "Full Foster" collapse position[66] where the runner crawls on elbows and knees and finally collapses before or after reaching the finish line. Regardless of the case, survival is threatened.

Here is another case. It is much less dramatic, but important for anybody who becomes fatigued while operating some machinery and for some reason cannot interrupt the process and rest. For example, pilots flying small airplanes face that problem.

Aviation

Decades ago, small airplanes didn't have autopilots since that option was hugely expensive. During those days, pilots didn't dare to nod off on long flights since the airplane might enter uncontrollable flight, for example, a deadly spiral.

Thus, the pilot combatted feelings of fatigue with powerful thoughts contemplating the consequences of closing the eyes.

Since then, innovative engineers have created low-cost autopilots for small airplanes, using compact electronics and electric motors. Thus, the plane can fly for an extended period without any pilot input, and nodding off has become tempting.

Suppose we are the pilot on one of those well-equipped airplanes. We are on a long trip, say consisting of two legs requiring four hours each.

As we feel fatigue coming on, we are tempted to reason, "Maybe I could close my eyes for a few seconds; it cannot possibly cause a problem." This is wrong, of course. Seconds may easily become minutes, with potentially disastrous consequences.

How can we fight this temptation? First, we might develop a training program where conscious thoughts modify subconscious neuroprocesses that output unjustified fatigue. CBT tells us that this will work.

But the solution doesn't sound very practical, does it?

Some time ago we learned about a different method that distracts the erroneous subconscious neuroprocesses.[67] When fatigue sets in, put a grape into your mouth, manipulate it for an extended period of several minutes, then bite on it, chew, and swallow. Repeat the process until the fatigue disappears.

It seems that the method works because each grape supplies a small sugar boost, which in turn helps overcome the fatigue. But is this the correct explanation? Maybe it's the manipulation of each grape in the mouth that plays the key role?

Indeed, subconscious neuroprocesses participate in the manipulation of each grape in the mouth and output the tactile sensation, the squashing of the grape, the chewing, and the sweet taste. That output pushes the fatigue output of other subconscious neuroprocesses into the background.

The method has one shortcoming. Each grape supplies not only sugar, but also some acid. Essentially, while this process goes on, the teeth are immersed in a slightly acidic bath. Not good for the tooth enamel, one would say.

Here is an alternative.[68] Instead of the grapes, you use nuts of a superior trail mix. There should be no raisins, peanuts, or sunflower seeds, just first-rate unsalted and roasted nuts such as almonds, cashews, pecan nuts, walnuts, macadamia nuts, and so on.

Pop one of the nuts into your mouth and swish it around. Use the teeth to gradually shave off some material. Keep on doing this until at some point the nut becomes soft and breaks up. Chew it carefully, and swallow.

This process takes about five minutes for each nut. The method does not introduce sugar or acid, but does supply a small amount of energy and also some fiber.

The process usually eliminates the fatigue within 15-20 minutes, thus requiring three to four nuts.

A simple solution, isn't it?

Temporary Replacement of Feelings

Do you see a major difference between the last case and every other situation we had discussed earlier? In the earlier ones, we relied on CBT to permanently change undesirable subconscious neuroprocesses.

The manipulation of nuts is different: We are aiming for a temporary elimination of the fatigue feeling, not for a permanent replacement. That's a good idea since fatigue messages generally protect our body from harm.

Some people don't want temporary elimination of fatigue and aim for permanent abolishment by thoughts and even chemistry, such as large amounts of coffee. It's a foolish attempt, of course. It terminates with one of two events. Either, the body truly caves in, for example, with a heart attack; or subconscious neuroprocesses produce a faked collapse in the form of panic attacks.[69]

The next chapter examines yet another case where subconscious neuroprocesses supply erroneous advice about our body.

12

Pain

When a minor injury prompts subconscious neuroprocesses to produce pain, we acknowledge the pain, examine the injury, and treat it appropriately. From then on, we generally avoid the pain, hoping that the body heals itself and the pain goes away.

Let's look at an example case where the reaction "Avoid the pain" fails badly.

Shoulder Injury

During the night, freezing rain has coated everything with a thin, almost invisible layer of ice. Not paying attention, John steps out in the morning to fetch the newspaper. He promptly slips, but breaks the fall with his right shoulder. Man, that hurts! He gets up and carefully shuffles back to the house.

He repeatedly applies an ice pack to the right shoulder, but the pain does not go away. He tells himself, "Don't move the shoulder" to avoid the pain, and goes on with life.

The next day, the pain sets in whenever he moves the shoulder to any significant extent. Hence he confines himself to small movements. The same happens the day after. In fact, the range of pain-less movement shrinks gradually. Eventually he cannot move the shoulder at all without significant pain. The shoulder has become *frozen.*

Evidently, the message "Don't move the shoulder" produced by subconscious neuroprocesses was wrong since it resulted in decisions and actions that ended up with a completely unusable shoulder. Why did evolution construct that mistaken response?

Explanation

When a hunter-gatherer hurt their shoulder, they could not stop looking for prey and plants and thus kept on moving the shoulder. Hence, "Avoid the pain" wasn't an option. Instead, they exercised the shoulder. It's only in modern times that "Avoid the pain" became a choice.

Seen in this light, evolution didn't make a mistake. It just didn't have enough time to create the correct response to such shoulder injuries for modern times.

It's easy to eliminate that maladaptive response. Every day, one exercises the full range of the shoulder movement with gentle movements that acknowledge the pain. While doing so, one should repeat the mantra "The pain is just a signal. I need to move the shoulder to promote healing." According to cognitive behavioral therapy (CBT), that self-talk changes the model of subconscious neuroprocesses issuing the pain and makes the pain more acceptable.

The remedial process becomes much more difficult once the shoulder has become frozen. A painful rehab program then requires weeks of exercises to gradually restore the range of movement.

Low Back Pain

The above situation is an instance of an entire class of pain situations where hunter-gatherers responded correctly by simply going on with their life and allowing the body to heal itself, and where a drastic change is needed in modern times. A prime example is low back pain.

At any given time, about 10% of the population experiences low back pain (LBP).[70] For example, lifting something heavy or a twisting movement or sharp bending forward may trigger low back pain the next day. Hunter-gatherers responded to the pain by going on with life. They carried out their daily tasks and thus exercised the back in multiple ways. That's exactly what one should do today. For example, yoga prescribes a wide range of exercises that aim to strengthen the back and eliminate the pain.

Instead, the afflicted person may take some pain killer and avoid movement involving the spine as much as possible. That virtually guarantees that the pain persists. The person then visits the family doctor and often enters an increasingly sophisticated treatment program.

In many if not most cases, yoga exercises over the next several weeks would produce the same if not better results.

Of course, there may be real damage that calls for complex treatment. But typically that is not the case.[71]

Pain and Pleasure

It turns out that the regions of the brain producing pain versus those generating feelings of pleasure overlap. Indeed, the two experiences are linked in the sense that subconscious neuroprocesses always try to achieve a neutral state. The appropriate image of the underlying model is a balance scale that goes down on the left when pleasure prevails, and descends on the right when pain is produced.[72]

The neuroprocesses try to keep the balance beam level. In particular, if drugs induce euphoria and thus depress the left-hand, or pleasure, side of the scale, then after a while there is a counter-reaction where that side rises again despite continued drug consumption. From then on, drugs are needed just to achieve a neutral response. Indeed, if drugs are then stopped, the right-hand side goes down and pain ensues. This is the withdrawal response after extended drug use.

Equally important: Suppose an injury produces pain. Hence, the right-hand side of the scale goes down. Without any drug use, that side later rises gradually and the pain slowly subsides. That happens in the above examples where exercising the shoulder or the entire body results in gradually subsiding pain.

If you want to learn more about the link connecting pain and pleasure, read the book *Dopamine Nation: Finding Balance in the Age of Indulgence*[73] by A. Lembke. It works out in detail how drugs interact and interfere with neuroprocesses, and how we can achieve an appropriate balance of pleasure and pain without drugs. The results can be readily restated in the terminology of models employed here. Indeed, the operation of a balancing scale connecting pain and pleasure is one such model.

The next chapter focuses on a general malaise of health care.

13

A Flood of Drugs

During the last 100 years science has produced numerous drugs that fight diseases once thought incurable. Many results seem almost miraculous, such as the obliteration of infections by antibiotics and the prevention of diseases by vaccines.

In recent decades, the use of drugs has been hugely expanded.[74]

- Doctors are flooded with drug samples and literature by the pharmaceutical industry, for short Pharma. This creates in their subconscious a web of models that propose drug treatment before anything else is considered.

  The effectiveness of the advertisements is limited since the doctor is unable to absorb all this material and incorporate it into his subconscious and conscious models for diagnosis.

  Pharma solves this problem by advertising their products to consumers in various media such as TV, newspapers, and magazines. This prods people with a particular disease to visit their doctor and ask for a prescription of the advertised drug.

- Pharma has managed to create a subconscious model in doctors that argues the following: Patients should be treated not only when ill, but also when they *may* become ill.

The combined effect: Subconscious models prod doctors to employ drugs for most illnesses, whether present or projected to occur in the future.

Let's look at three examples.

Fentanyl

The opioid Fentanyl is likely the most abused yet legal drug. Synthesized in 1958 and approved for medical use in the US in 1968, it was intended for pain management. Since it is 50 to 100 times more potent than morphine, it was prescribed for the most severe situations such as for cancer patients and after painful surgical operations.[75]

Unscrupulously produced in vast quantities and supplied by irresponsible prescriptions, Fentanyl has fueled an epidemic of synthetic opioid deaths in the US. Just in 2021, Fentanyl caused more than 70,000 overdose deaths.

There is little that you, by yourself, can do about this. But you can exercise control when you suffer from significant pain and look at Fentanyl as a treatment option. The advice: "Don't rely on it." Fentanyl is highly addictive when taken for any extended period. Instead, work on the pain, and if possible, solve the problem by non-drug treatment. A change of subconscious models by cognitive behavioral therapy (CBT) can be most helpful when coupled with appropriate physical therapy. For example, low back pain can often be resolved that way; see Chapter 12.

Fosamax

The strength of bones in the body derives from calcium held in the bones. When the calcium is gradually depleted, bones lose their strength and may deform and break. That awful process is called osteoporosis.[76]

As men and women age, osteoporosis often sets in, as is evident in any old folks home where bent-over men and women shuffle with a walker in the hallways.

What can be done about this debilitating disease? Well, the first line of defense is not getting it in the first place.

Sounds silly, doesn't it? But the statement is correct. Lifestyle has a huge impact on the loss of calcium. Here are seven steps to avoid that disaster:[77]

- Have a healthy and varied diet with plenty of fresh fruit, vegetables and whole grains.
- Eat calcium-rich foods.
- Absorb enough vitamin D.
- Avoid smoking.
- Limit alcohol consumption.
- Limit caffeine.
- Do regular weight-bearing and strength-training activities.

You may quibble about what "Avoid smoking" or "Limit alcohol consumption" mean. But there is no mistaking the last demand of weight-bearing and strength-training. It requires a determined effort every day or at least several times a week.

We know this since the astronauts—a select group of people in excellent physical condition—lose calcium in space since their zero weight removes all stress on the bones.[78]

Pharma created an easily adopted alternative: the drug Fosamax, generic name alendronic acid. It promised to stop the depletion of calcium and thus prevent or stop osteoporosis. The drug was first described in 1978. It was approved for medical use in the US in 1995.

In 2020, doctors prescribed Fosamax 7 million times, making the drug the 94th most commonly prescribed medication in the US.

That success was only possible due to another development: low-cost measurement of bone density.

The invention of Dual-Energy X-ray Absorptiometry (DEXA) in the 1980s made this possible.[79] Any doctor's office could install a DEXA machine. The result: Doctors measured bone density even when there was no indication that a test was needed. This paved the way for the flood of Fosamax prescriptions.

Here are some of the serious side effects of Fosamax:[80]

- Peptic ulcer and possible rupture of the esophagus

- Cancer of the esophagus

- Osteonecrosis of the jaw, where the blood flow to the jaw is disrupted and the bone tissue breaks down

- Low-impact femoral fractures

- An increase in the number of osteoclasts, which are bone cells that break down bone tissue

Shouldn't everyone prefer to change lifestyle instead of taking Fosamax and potentially suffer debilitating side effects?

That decision requires a change of subconscious models. Instead of output such as "I don't need to worry, Fosamax will take care of the problem," we must create a model that outputs positive feelings about the change of lifestyle.

What does all this mean for you? The following seems prudent.

- Engage in a lifestyle that prevents the loss of calcium in the bones.

- Do not use any osteoporosis drug, such as Fosamax, as a preventative measure.

- If you are in a high-risk group for the disease, monitor bone density with periodic tests and stay updated about treatments.

Obesity Drugs

As we saw in Chapter 9, obesity rates in the US more than tripled from 13% of adults in 1960 to 42% in 2022.[81]

The chapter also argues that ever-increasing consumption of optimized foods and drinks is a key cause of that dramatic rise.

An appropriate reaction would focus on drastic reduction of that consumption, as described earlier. That hasn't happened. Instead, Pharma has created a monstrous drug program where every obese person is supposed to take some medication for the rest of their lives.

There are various drugs on the market, and more to come.[82] Given the limited time they have been used, we do not have a thorough understanding of the long-term consequences.

But from the drug trials and use to date, we are already aware of short-term complications. For example, for the blockbuster anti-obesity drug Wegovy, we know about the following, very serious side effects:[83]

- Low blood sugar in people with type 2 diabetes
  Symptoms can include dizziness, sweating, and confusion.
- Pancreatitis (inflammation of the pancreas)
  Symptoms can include abdominal pain, fever, nausea, and vomiting.
- Gallbladder problems
  Symptoms can include abdominal pain, nausea, and vomiting
- Kidney problems
  Symptoms can include urinating more or less often than is typical, nausea, vomiting, and fatigue.
- Diabetic eye problems
  Symptoms can include blurry vision and vision loss.
- Depression or suicidal thoughts or behavior
- Increased heart rate

- Risk of thyroid cancer
- Severe allergic reaction

If aliens were visiting the earth, they would conclude the following. The humans consume vast amounts of optimized foods. It causes an addiction to food, overeating, and eventually obesity. The people of the earth have decided to ignore this connection and instead have created drugs that combat obesity with significant side effects, not to mention extraordinary cost.[84]

We could go on and discuss other drugs that can be avoided, often are harmful and nearly always expensive, sometimes obscenely so. But this would serve little purpose here.

After all, our goal isn't to lament the greed of Pharma since there is nothing you or I can do about it. Instead, we look in the next chapter at decisions you can make so you don't have to take these drugs in the first place.

14

Alternatives

There is no doubt that a diet based on optimized foods, as described in Chapter 8, is virtually guaranteed to result in severe illnesses. Doctors try to prevent them with drugs that, for example, lower cholesterol and blood pressure, or suppress appetite. Going that route, it seems that you can both eat the seductive food and maintain your health.

That is a delusion, as you discover as you get older. For example, you may start to suffer from depression or insomnia. But the doctor has drugs for those problems, too.

Eventually you become a major consumer of various drugs, some with nasty side effects. What started out as a deceptively simple and appealing solution has turned into a train wreck.

Why not avoid that process and its complications altogether? Here's how.

First and foremost, you must avoid optimized foods, just as an alcoholic must give up all alcohol consumption. Chapter 9 describes how you can do this.

But there is more. Now and then your body will act up, so to speak. Your subconscious may well put out the unbidden thought "Let's go and visit our family doctor or a specialist." After all, that's what you have health insurance for, haven't you? If you accept that argument, you will see your doctor or a specialist right away and start taking some drugs that often do, but sometimes don't, cure the problem. In either case, the drugs may produce nasty side effects.

Rational Reaction

A wiser approach is the following. You respond to the subconscious unbidden thought with the conscious "Let's first find out something about the problem." Following that different path, you inform yourself about steps you can take to alleviate if not cure the problem while avoiding the use of drugs altogether. That becomes your goal.

A key source for information is the Internet. Yes, it produces lots and lots of untrustworthy information. But it also connects you with reliable sources.

For example, the *People's Pharmacy* offers a wealth of material covering simple and effective treatment of numerous illnesses and afflictions.[85]

Numerous books offer helpful information, too.

An example: The book *How Not to Die: Discover the Foods Scientifically Proven to Prevent and Reserve Disease*[86] by M. Greger discusses foods that are extraordinarily helpful. The book covers fifteen major illnesses, ranging from heart, lung, and brain diseases to infections and several cancers. Part II of the book lists how specific foods help, ranging from beans, berries, and other fruits to whole grains, herbs, and spices.

Of course, your investigation may turn up that you should see a doctor, or may even urge you to hurry to the nearest hospital. But those decisions are based on a rational investigation and not on the unbidden thought "Let's go and visit our family doctor or a specialist." In fact, once you have had the rational thought "Let's first find out something about the problem" several times, your subconscious changes and offers it as the first reaction.

Folk Medicine

Asian and European folk medicines include numerous treatment teas and other simple remedies. Unfortunately, the advertising flood by Pharma has pushed much of that information into oblivion. But determined searches on the Internet still find relevant information. Here is one example.

Kidney stones can cause extraordinary pain when they move from the kidneys to the bladder. How can one prevent them? The typical recommendation includes drinking lots of fluids, reducing salt intake, and avoiding excessive calcium intake. A bit more difficult to find is the following age-old European recommendation: Prevent or treat kidney stones by drinking one cup of tea brewed with goldenrod every day.[87]

Summary

The protection of your body from the ills caused by inappropriate foods and medicines requires a determined effort on all fronts. Whenever you are about to ingest some food or medication, you should ask yourself, "Is this good for me?" like a mantra.

In many cases, you conclude that you should reject that food or medicine, and look for a different, healthier alternative.

When you seemingly suffer from some ailment, follow the mantra "Let's first find out something about the problem" and investigate via the Internet.

Many cases will turn out to be a minor nuisance that you can deal with on your own. Others will prompt a visit to your doctor. You may even identify a calamity where you must rush to the nearest hospital.

After a while, the deliberate process becomes ingrained and part of a simpler and healthier lifestyle.

The Romans had the saying *Mens sana in corpore sano* (A healthy mind in a healthy body). We have covered the *corpore sano* portion of the adage. In the next part, we investigate the *mens sana* goal.

Part II

Mind

15
Mind Definition

"Mind" has been defined in numerous ways. This includes an overall, vague declaration that mind is the collection of all faculties involved in mental phenomena.[88]

Our definition in this book allows for two distinct cases and relies on the interpretation of statements such as "In my mind, we should ...," (= "In my *thinking*, we should ...") and "Please keep in mind that ...," (= "Please be *aware* that ...").

The first statement refers to the activities of the conscious neuroprocesses, while the second one focuses on our awareness of them.

The following definition captures both cases and expands upon an earlier characterization.[89]

> *Mind* refers to the activities of the conscious neuroprocesses as well as our awareness of them. The latter case includes awareness of the feelings and unbidden thoughts supplied by the subconscious neuroprocesses to the conscious ones.

You may wonder: Why do we introduce the new term "mind" when we have already the concept of conscious neuroprocesses and use the fact that we are aware of them? The reason: In this part, we frequently refer to the conscious neuroprocesses and our awareness of them. The term "mind" compactly refers to both cases.

The effects of erroneous subconscious output on our mind are far ranging. For example, the faulty output may induce us to adopt wrong investment strategies, propel us to spend endless hours traversing the Internet, or push us to overtax our body so badly that it goes on strike.

The causes for that erroneous output are just as diverse. For the three examples: A niggling wish for adventure is part of daring investment strategies, a natural curiosity makes us spend endless hours on the Internet, and an impatient drive to reach difficult goals leads to the abuse of the body.

As we shall see, these causes are rooted in features of the subconscious neuroprocesses that worked well in the distant past for hunter-gatherers, but are no longer appropriate today. That insight guides us when we eliminate these problems.

Needless to say, it's beyond our powers to provide a comprehensive treatment. But just as in the case of the body, the specific cases we do discuss should help you develop general skills to recognize harmful situations, identify root causes, and come up with effective solutions.

We begin with a practical question: How should we plan financially for retirement?

16

A Dead-Sure Investor

Here is a true story about an investor and his strategies, except that the names have been changed.

Strategy 1: Buy and Sell Stocks

John is a successful engineer. Early on, a stock broker advises that John should invest his savings in stocks. John agrees and starts to purchase shares on the broker's recommendations. The portfolio grows to a nice sum. John is proud of his achievement. He is building wealth the right way.

But then the market retreats. In particular, one stock in John's portfolio tanks. John thinks, "This is just one small bump in the road." The stock broker recommends that John sell that stock and reinvest the money in another stock. This should fix the problem, John thinks.

Further market losses reduce the portfolio even more. John sees his investments melt away and becomes upset. How can he salvage the portfolio?

He decides on a daring attempt to make up for all those losses. He sells everything except for one stock, where he invests everything.

According to his broker, that stock is sure to become a blowout success.

He discusses his decision with friend Richard, who responds, "This is not a good idea. You are running a substantial risk of failure." But John trusts the broker. After all, he is an expert, isn't he?

The market declines even further. Worse yet, the selected company goes bankrupt. All savings are gone. John is devastated. How could this disaster happen? John has just one explanation: Rapid buying and selling of stocks is a mistake. He will never do that again.

Strategy 2: Buy and Hold Stocks

It's many years later. John now works for a large and successful high-tech company. Using a company-sponsored investment plan, he buys stock in his company. On top, he invests whatever money is left at the end of each month in the same stock.

He keeps on buying regardless of the movement of the market. His mantra is "I just count the number of shares." It is the opposite of his earlier strategy, where he bought and sold stocks. John is dead certain that this is the correct method for investment success.

An almost catastrophic market collapse tests the mettle of investors. In the turmoil John clings to his mantra and holds on to the large number of shares he has accumulated. He says, "This is just temporary, and it will all work out." Sure enough, the market recovers rapidly, confirming John's prediction. John is elated. Finally he has the right formula for success. The quick recovery from the losses proves it.

By now, John has amassed stock worth two million dollars. Effectively, he is done with saving for retirement. By switching to a conservative investment plan, he would be financially secure for the rest of his life.

But John feels that things will get even better and continues with his strategy. Talking it over with Richard, the friend advises, "Why don't you sell half of the shares and place the proceeds in a secure investment?"

John recalls how he held firm when the market collapsed, and how quickly the market recovered. Clearly, putting half of the investment in some humdrum safe storage means that he will miss out on substantial future profits. Why do this when he has the right formula for success?

The earnings of his company decline slowly. Even though the market rises, the price of his stock goes gradually down. Once more Richard advises selling half of the portfolio. John feels that he has come so far, and that many times the stock went down a bit and then recovered. He decides to make no change, and responds, "I will do this once the stock price has recovered."

The price keeps on declining. John argues that all this is temporary and that the stock will recover. Eventually, the price drops to 16% of the peak value. He has lost almost all of his retirement savings. He panics and sells everything.[90]

Right at that time, the company hires a new CEO who tries to grow the profit by laying off senior employees. This includes John. He now is out of a job, too.

Strategy 3: Take Lump Sum Instead of Pension

The company offers him a pension or, alternately, a lump sum payment. The pension looks so small compared with the lump sum. John thinks that the pension is just a promise of future payments, while the lump sum is here and now. Doing a quick computation, he concludes that he can do much better with the lump sum than the promised pension.

Richard advises, "Go for the pension. It will be a guaranteed part of your retirement income." John declines, "I can do much better if I invest the lump sum." John intuitively feels that it would be exciting to beat the pension plan.

John puts some of the proceeds into the safe investments recommended by Richard. But he also identifies a money manager who guarantees a 12% return for a totally safe investment. A key financial publication praises the manager. John decides to invest much of the remaining money to reap that amazing return.

John discusses his decision with Richard, who cautions him, "Don't do this! A 12% return on investment must entail substantial risk." Richard even gives a short lecture why high returns must entail a significant probability that the investment will fail. If that wasn't so, everyone would invest for the high return, and offers with lower return would disappear.

The argument doesn't impress John. He repeats that the past performance of the manager has been terrific. The popular financial publication has said so.

The supposedly safe investment program turns out to be a house of cards. The investments crash, and John loses everything. The final result: After 40 years of investing, John has accumulated a paltry amount.

Explanation

John evidently deluded himself that he knew how to invest. In the process, he committed blunder after blunder. Why would he do that, and persist even when a knowledgeable friend counseled the opposite?

Deep down in the subconscious is the drive to take chances. Evolution installed that urge since a hunter-gatherer who explored new things had better chances of survival. Evolution also constructed a subconscious trust that we can, indeed should, predict what will happen next.

The investment industry exploits these two features of the subconscious neuroprocesses. Agents lay out convincingly why some investments are far superior to others. The business section of newspapers, numerous financial magazines, and several financial TV channels reinforce this belief. Yes, there is risk, but then, did anybody ever get anywhere without assuming some risk?

———————————

The next chapter lays out in detail how the investment industry exploits the subconscious drive for exciting new investment actions and the belief in financial predictions.

17

Bad Advice

Suppose you want to invest in the stock market, but are a novice. Naively you search the Internet for "stock investment advice."[91] The search produces many sites, each offering different suggestions. Yet each site claims that their choice maximizes portfolio growth. Confusing, isn't it? How should you proceed?

Maybe you shouldn't try to do this on your own and instead should engage a financial advisor. Let's see how that would work out.

The advisor generally suggests that you acquire individual stocks or shares in a mutual fund. In the latter case, some corporation has acquired stock of a number of companies, and you buy shares of that collection.

The advisor generally gets paid in one of two ways: through a portion of the money involved in the transactions or through a yearly fee, typically 1% of your portfolio.

In the first case, the advisor makes suggestions that maximize their income. Stock brokers fall into this category. They earn commissions when you buy and sell. Hence the broker recommends that you buy and sell frequently.

This may include truly bad proposals, for example, the suggestion that you invest in a mutual fund with high management fees and a front-end load charge, followed some time later by the recommendation that you move to another mutual fund and repeat the costly process.

Regardless of the situation, the following image is appropriate: You are hiring a fox to guard the hen house.[92]

In the second case, the fee charged by the advisor is an added cost burden for the investment that significantly reduces the growth of the portfolio.

You may be surprised by our harsh criticism. But it is justified. The advisor really doesn't know more than you do, in the sense that they do not have a crystal ball to predict the future. It's just that they act as if they do. That façade plays into models of your subconscious neuroprocesses where opinions of experts are accompanied with the unbidden thought that they really know and can be trusted.

Particularly bad investment decisions are next.

18

Mistakes

Some investments are bound to fail. Here are important cases.

Investment in Individual Stocks

Nobody knows which stocks will rise and which will decline. In particular, nobody can predict where new technology will take us and thus which stocks will become winners.

For example, who would have guessed a few decades ago the following:

- The cell phone connects us with family, friends, indeed the world.

- More than two billion computers[93] are tied together in a network with enormous transmission capacity. The system supplies virtually all information worldwide.

- Computing is universal in the sense that powerful chips are embedded in virtually every device. Even wristwatches have begun to contain them.

Why would you be tempted to invest in individual stocks? The financial news tout almost daily that some company has produced incredible earnings and that the stock price is rising rapidly.

Subconscious neuroprocesses produce the unbidden thought "I wish I had bought that stock." That thought plays into the hands of advisors who claim to know how to select winners.

Suppose you sign up and buy on their advice. Generally, this doesn't work out well.

But whenever your portfolio runs into headwinds, the advisor has an appropriate explanation and offers new suggestions for buying and selling. This can go on for years without you ever realizing that ownership of individual stocks is a mistake.

Investment in the Company Where You Work

If the company offers stock at a reduced cost as part of profit sharing, do buy the stock, but sell it again as soon as the rules permit.

There is a strong temptation to hang on to such stock, and possibly buy even more outside the company plan. You mistakenly think that you have deep insight into the company's operation and can predict its financial future.

Indeed, whenever there is some news, you feel that you know that already from your work. This creates the unbidden thought "I fully understand what is going on here," which makes investing in company shares look like a slam dunk for success.

But when the company falls upon hard times, top management hides this from you as long as possible. Since you erroneously believe that you understand everything about the company, you interpret a declining stock price as a temporary phenomenon, when in reality the market anticipates poor financial performance. Hence instead of selling, you hang on to the stock and incur ever increasing losses.

If the stock tanks, you may also be laid off at a time when you can least afford it.

Supposedly Safe Investment With High Return

High return and zero risk are fundamentally incompatible. For example, the investment may be part of a Ponzi scheme where initial investors are paid using the contributions of subsequent ones,[94] or the investments have a hidden high risk of failure.[95]

Rejecting high-return offers is difficult since the rosy promise triggers a warm and fuzzy response by subconscious neuroprocesses. At the same time, you have no way to account for the risk. In fact, as far as you are able to determine, there is no risk. But there *is* risk. You just don't know the details.

The investor of Chapter 16 made every one of these bad choices, in part under the guidance of an advisor. How can we avoid them, yet invest in the stock market? Let's see.

19

Solution

Mankind has achieved miraculous success using a plethora of models. Based on them, we fly to the moon; cure horrible diseases; and build computers, houses, cars, railroads, and airplanes. It's an almost endless list of wondrous achievements.

This huge success is reflected in our subconscious neuroprocesses. When they receive information about a problem, they send not just the problem formulation to the conscious neuroprocesses, but also supply feelings and unbidden thoughts that we should employ models for the solution.

This automatic response serves us well when the construction of conscious models indeed can help us. But it misguides us when unbeknownst to us a model for the solution of our problem most likely doesn't exist.

Picking stocks is a problem of the latter kind. Though many people believe that they can build a detailed selection model, the reality is that this can't be done by anybody, including experts in finance.

How do we know this? It's evident from the fact that everyone who claimed to have a model for selecting stocks failed to produce good results consistently.

What are we to do? The answer involves two steps.

- We must learn how to invest in a certain way that is virtually guaranteed to produce good if not excellent results. The idea underlying the approach is very different from anything we have seen so far. The basic idea is so unusual that the inventor of the approach was ridiculed when he first proposed it. But in 2023, more than 10 trillion dollars were invested that way with outstanding results, and nobody is laughing anymore.

- We must learn to reject any other investment scheme. We can do this with conscious thoughts that modify subconscious models.

When we have completed both steps, we can invest with confidence that the investments will grow and achieve our goals. That confidence eliminates the stress typically connected with investments. Indeed, we have abandoned the futile hunt for gold at the end of a rainbow and are ready to enjoy life.

Let's look at details of the two steps.

First Step: How to Invest

The US economy grows yearly at a certain rate. On average, the stock market grows along with it. Why not invest in the entire market and thus consistently partake in that long-term growth?

Based on this idea, John C. Bogle pioneered the world's first *index fund* in 1976.[96]

The fund simultaneously invests in the 500 largest companies of the US. It is called the *S&P 500 Index Fund* since it relies on the Standard and Poor 500 Index. We look at details in a moment.

It is impossible to overstate the importance of Bogle's invention. The economist Paul Samuelson placed it at the same level as the invention of the wheel, the alphabet, and Gutenberg printing.[97]

What was Bogle's idea? It's easiest to understand via a simplified example. Suppose a stock exchange lists just two companies called

Big and Small. Shares of the two companies are bought and sold every day.

When we multiply the total number of outstanding shares of Big with the current share price, we get Big's *market capitalization*. The same applies to Small. When we add the two market capitalization values, we get the *total market capitalization* for the exchange. Let's abbreviate that to *total market*. That value goes up or down virtually every day, depending on the price of the two stocks.

Bogle invented how we can invest in Big and Small so that our investment moves exactly like the total market. Well, not in absolute numbers, but percentagewise. So if the total market goes up or down by, say, 20%, our investment matches that percentage change.

Let's look at an example how we can accomplish this. Suppose Big's market capitalization is $700,000 and that of Small $300,000. Hence the total market is $700,000 + $300,000 = $1,000,000.

Suppose we want to invest $100,000. That is, we want to invest $100,000/1,000,000 = 10\%$ of the total market. We then buy shares of Big so that their value is equal to 10% of Big's market capitalization $700,000. That's $70,000. Correspondingly, we buy 10% of Small's market capitalization $300,000, which is $30,000. Together, we have invested $100,000 as desired.

Suppose the market goes up by 20%. No matter how share prices of Big and Small change to produce this effect, our portfolio changes by 20% as well. That's due to the fact that our portfolio is nothing but a scaled version of the market. In some sense it *tracks the market*.

Let's apply this to the companies of the S&P 500 index. The numbers are much bigger, of course, but the principle is the same. There is a glitch, though. If an investor were to implement the above scheme, they would have to buy shares of 500 companies each time they invest. That's completely impractical.

Here is Bogle's solution. Vanguard, the company founded by Bogle, acquires stock of the 500 companies as described. Vanguard then allocates the purchase to investors. This process can be done daily.

Say, today several thousand investors place orders for purchases with Vanguard. Overnight, Vanguard collates the orders and arrives at a total purchase amount. The next day, Vanguard purchases stock for that total purchase amount and credits the account of each investor with the appropriate portion. Voilá, the investment of each investor moves percentagewise exactly like the S&P 500 index.

When Bogle first proposed index investing in 1976, the method was ridiculed since the investment choices didn't involve any evaluation of company performance. Surely cleverly selected purchases could do much better. It turned out that the criticism was quite wrong. Vanguard's S&P 500 Index Fund typically has outperformed 80 to 90% of all mutual funds.

How is this possible? There are three reasons.

- The professionals who supposedly understand how the market works and which companies will succeed, often are mistaken in their belief.

- Vanguard's costs of operation are minute compared with the large expenses associated with mutual funds. For example, Vanguard charges 0.04% per year for larger portfolios. Suppose you have a portfolio of $500,000. Then the 0.04% yearly cost is $200, which is almost nothing compared with the $4,000 to $5,000 charge of a typical mutual fund.

- There is a subtle but important aspect of the index fund. If the performance of a company in the index declines as measured by market capitalization and becomes less than that of a company outside the index, the corporation[98] maintaining the S&P 500 index replaces the smaller company with the newcomer.

Vanguard carries out the same swap with appropriate buying and selling. As a result, the fund automatically tracks changes of technology in the sense that it always invests correctly when new ideas take root.

This became very much evident during the last 30 years. That period spawned technology giants such as Apple, Alphabet, Amazon, and Microsoft. When these companies entered the S&P 500 index, investors in the index fund automatically acquired ownership in those companies.

Much more can be said about index funds. There are funds for segments of the stock market, for example defined by capitalization or by fields of endeavor such as health care.

There is even an index fund for the entire US stock market. Other index funds cover foreign stock markets, bonds, and real estate. It is a plethora of offerings.[99]

How do you select from this palette of investment possibilities? Some people suggest that you partition your portfolio and invest separately in several index funds. Others counsel simple approaches, for example, segmenting your portfolio into two portions for stocks and bonds, and then use two index funds.

Our opinion: Keep it simple and do not move in and out of index funds in the mistaken belief that you know better. Like individual stock purchases, such swaps are a futile chase of gold at the end of the rainbow.

There is a philosophical aspect. Bogle always believed that investors large and small should achieve their goals with minimal expense, and that the sole purpose of the personnel of Vanguard, from top to bottom, was working toward that objective. The employees receive appropriate salaries, but there is no hidden incentive to make money off investors. In effect, the investors are the owners of Vanguard, and Vanguard's employees work for them.[100]

Second Step: How to Reject Tempting Choices

At this point, we know how to invest. But what about our feelings about the investments? Won't financial news about incredibly successful companies and their rapidly rising stocks create regretful and wishful thoughts? Won't we feel left behind with our indexing method and regret that we didn't select booming stocks instead?

If we accept these errant feelings and unbidden thoughts of subconscious neuroprocesses, we become unhappy every day since there is always some very successful company.

Cognitive behavioral theory (CBT) advises us how to eliminate these negative feelings and unbidden thoughts, as follows. Every time we see rosy news about some company, we consciously think:

- "This is just daily noise. What matters are the next 10 and 20 years. Nobody knows where this company will end up."

- "If that company is truly outstanding, one of two things will happen. Either the company will be bought by some company already in the S&P 500 index or eventually will enter that index by itself. Regardless of the case, I will automatically own part of that company."[101]

You summarize this with a daily mantra:

My index investments capture the advances of successful companies. There is no need for me to get involved in individual stocks.

Vanguard has reduced this to the following advice:

Stay the course.

If you repeat these thoughts and mantras every day, negative emotions and unbidden thoughts triggered by financial news begin to recede into the background and eventually disappear. At that time, reading those news will become as important as, say, learning about the weather in some country far away. It is information but doesn't mean anything for your well-being.

Sometimes you may hear the advice "Do invest in index funds, but also keep a very small portfolio of individual stocks you buy and sell. That way, you can pursue supposedly excellent opportunities. When those stocks tank, there is little harm done to your wealth."

The advice is similar to advising an alcoholic to stay sober, but indulge in a small amount of alcohol every day nevertheless. It's not good advice for the alcoholic just as the counsel of a small handpicked portfolio is a bad idea.

If your selected stocks perform worse than the index, you feel sad since you could have done better.

If by sheer luck your stocks outperform the index investment during a given year, you feel sad that you didn't invest all your money in handpicked stocks. There is no way to win, is there?

On the other hand, if you rely on indexing for everything, you sleep at night and during the day can focus on your life.

Once your investment program has born sufficient fruit for comfortable support in later years, you may want to think about others that are worse off than you are. How can you help them with a long-term program? Let's see.

Helping Others

You can assist folks that are far worse off than you via a charitable fund that you create and control. You can do so, for example, by opening an account with Vanguard Charitable.

You supply the start-up funding and direct that it is invested in the S&P 500 index fund. Technically, you do not own the investment. But you do have full control over its management.

The dividend return for that fund is about 2% per year. Hence, every year you direct 2% of the fund to be distributed to organizations that help folks much less fortunate than you. The fund will still grow due to capital gains. You do not pay income tax on the dividends or the capital gains since you do not own the fund.

As the years roll by, the fund becomes larger and larger. Correspondingly, the 2% disbursement grows as well. It is a self-sustaining and automatically growing venture. It will go on forever if you direct your heirs to continue the management and they pass it on to their heirs, and so on. How nice!

Harmful Optimization

There is another way to look at the devious efforts of much of the investment industry. Using advertising, newspaper articles, specialized publications, and TV programs, these companies have created a make-believe world for investing.

The goal is extracting a huge amount of money from investors, all under the guise of investment advice. We call this an *optimized investment strategy* since it maximizes profits for the investment companies. At the same time, the strategy results in extraordinary harm for investors. One of the rare exceptions is the Vanguard Company, which effectively is owned by and solely works for the investors.

We have seen a similarly devious effort in Chapter 8: The food industry has created *optimized foods* that maximize profits by luring people into ever-increasing consumption of addiction-forming foods.

The next chapter covers the devious optimization process of yet another industry. It, too, aims to maximize profits. The strategy inflicts extraordinary damage on people.

20

Digital Media

Humans have created a wondrous world of communication: We send texts, photos, even videos to anybody around the globe without charge. We access libraries online and read books published in the distant past. We get answers for almost any question via living encyclopedias that are updated daily. We stream movies and listen to podcasts covering a vast range of topics. With a single click, we find efficient driving routes. We read online newspapers that are updated several times a day.

Digital media makes this possible, and much more. Amazing, isn't it?

Yet, there is a dark side to this information bonanza: We become so addicted to the flood of offerings that we spend hours every day receiving and sending information.

On top, some of the information we soak up changes us in fundamental ways, to the point where any alien visiting the earth would conclude that effectively we have ceded much control over our lives to machines. This is particularly so for social media.

You may object that this is a vast exaggeration. If so, you may want to read the book *The Chaos Machine: The Inside Story of How Social Media Rewired Our Minds and Our World*[102] by M. Fisher.

It not only describes the devious processes by which social media pushes people to pursue information and thus go down ever deeper rabbit holes, but also lays out the horrific consequences.

For example, Facebook spread wild conspiracy theories that fueled the genocide of the minority Muslim Rohingya of Myanmar.[103] At least 25,000 were killed, tens of thousands raped, and more than 700,000 fled abroad.[104]

In the US, social media has triggered pathological computer use, eating disorders, social anxiety, lowered self-esteem, and even suicide.[105]

How can we prevent these disasters? Two steps: First, we work out why and how digital media draw us in. Second, we learn to avoid the parts of digital media that damage us.

The book *Digital Minimalism: Choosing a Focused Life in a Noisy World*[106] by C. Newport describes both steps in impressive detail. We shall not attempt to duplicate that exposition. But we include a summarizing description that also relies on the incisive book *Dopamine Nation: Finding Balance in the Age of Indulgence*[107] by A. Lembke. The latter book uses recent results of neuroscience to establish the causes of addiction, then proposes powerful remedies.

The next chapter summarizes the devious processes of some digital media.

21

Economics and Evolution

Digital media relies on a range of methods for financial support.

At one end are organizations that now and then ask for a voluntary contribution or require modest subscription fees for their service. Wikipedia[108] and the Internet Archive[109] fall into this category. They provide extraordinary services, operate on very limited funding, and have no detrimental impact on the user. Other examples are electronic versions of traditional newspapers with a history of reliable reporting, for example, The New York Times.[110]

At the other end are organizations like Facebook[111] and Twitter[112] that rely on a sophisticated, indirect method to produce earnings. We call them *profit-driven digital media* and abbreviate this to *profit media*.

In between is digital media that on the surface operates in a benign manner, but deep down also contributes to the malaise created by profit media. It nominally imposes no charges on the user, but actually collects, uses, or sells information, for example, for targeted advertising. Examples are the search engines Google[113] and Bing.[114]

In this chapter we examine the underpinnings of profit media.

Advertising

Business makes money by selling products or providing services. In the olden days, business advertised in a broad-brush approach where most recipients of ads weren't even remotely interested in the offerings.

Profit media has replaced this ineffective method with a sophisticated approach. Depending on the view, the scheme either is a wonderful result of capitalism since it creates huge profits, or is a devilish machinery that relies on an economic domestication of the users.

What does "economic domestication" mean?

Let's see.

Domestication

Humans wouldn't have been able to dominate the world without the domestication of animals such as horses, camels, llamas, oxen, cows, pigs, sheep, dogs, cats, and chickens. Once humans achieved this, these animals helped to plant, harvest, and process food; construct buildings; pump water; tow carts and boats; and on and on. Also, some of the domesticated animals produced food, helped with hunting of other animals, or became themselves food.

The domesticated animals freed up humans to think about things other than just food, clothing, and shelter. For example, they had time to build machines, develop cures for diseases, and develop the sciences.

We see an analogous development today that, in contrast, isn't beneficial for us but outright horrendous. It involves another kind of domestication where we, the people of the earth, are being domesticated by profit media. Indeed, we are being manipulated into actions that have two effects: They produce huge profits for that media, and they are extraordinarily harmful for us.

We aren't alone with that view. The book *Digital Minimalism: Choosing a Focused Life in a Noisy* World[115] by C. Newport talks about the "feeling of *losing control*" and says, "[W]e were *pushed* into [a digital life we didn't sign up for]."

How did profit media accomplish this?

Economics

Profit media has turned the construction and delivery of ads into a devilish clever process that, well, domesticates the user. Here are the steps.

First, profit media collects vast amounts of information about each person wherever and whenever possible. For example, they record which books and newspapers we read, what TV channels we watch, what Internet sites we visit, where we go out to eat, and what we purchase where. Supposedly benign digital media such as the search engines Google and Bing takes part in this collection effort.

Based on that information, profit media offers numerous tailored ads that, for example, prod us to purchase some food, buy a dress or coat, watch a certain movie, read some book, or acquire a new car.

The targeted ads wouldn't be effective if we wouldn't look at them. Profit media overcomes this constraint by inducing us to stay connected as long as possible. It accomplishes this using an innate drive created by evolution and refined over millennia: Curiosity. The German term "Neugierde" captures the gist of this drive: We have an inherent greed ("Gierde") for new ("neu") information.

Greed for New Information

During the several million years of human development, humans faced ever changing conditions. Anybody who ignored these changes was more likely to die earlier than the folks who paid attention to the changes and adapted accordingly. In fact, babies grow and eventually become mature adults only if they are receptive to new information, investigate the sources, and adapt.

There is another way to state this: Humans have inborn subconscious models that trigger an investigation whenever something new shows up.

Activating and Maintaining the Greed

Two factors determine the amount of time the user spends on profit media: How often the user uses it, and how long they stay connected each time. Media maximizes both factors by exploiting the evolution-created greed for new information.

This takes several forms, but the principle behind each of them is the same: The setting entices the user to link up with media and then stay there for an extended period.

For example, when a user has posted a message on Facebook for their friends, they feel compelled to check time and again for "like" responses, then get lured to read additional information, respond to it, and so on. Or media offers enticing images with suggestive titles, such as "Her Dress Left Little to the Mind's Eye."

Even more devious are images and text that, according to the background amassed about a user, are sure to rile them up. The discomfort, even anger, raised by the information triggers an extended dive into a never-ending rabbit hole.

YouTube uses yet another method. When the user has just finished viewing a video, YouTube suggests a next, related video, and then yet another one, and so on. Youtube may also propose videos that aren't really connected with the ones already shown, but maximize the odds that the user will view them and dive down yet another rabbit hole.

A seemingly innocuous feature called *continuous* or *infinite scroll* enables the user to scroll endlessly down a page that may be arbitrarily long. That feature hides from the user how much time they are spending on the page since they just read on and on.

In contrast, if they had to click for additional pages, it would be a reminder that they are committing an extraordinary amount of time to the website and should stop.

In 2021, these methods and, yes, tricks caused users to spend more than eight hours every day on digital media. Of course, that number includes useful connect time, for example, searches for some information, translations, processing important messages, and so on. But there is another, truly alarming number. During 2023, users spent 2-3 hours each day on social media such as Facebook, YouTube, WhatsApp, Instagram, Facebook Messenger, and TikTok.

How can we escape these devious processes? We see next how we can reach this difficult goal.

22

Escape From Profit Media

The addiction to profit media is as difficult to cure as alcoholism or smoking.

Just watch people waiting to board a plane at the airport, sitting in a doctor's waiting room, attending a ball game, waiting for a train to arrive or a theatre performance to start, or being at home with supposedly nothing to do.

Regardless of the case, most people ignore their surroundings, hypnotized by the small screen of their smartphone.

If you focus on one person, you notice that they look at the screen, scroll and maybe tap for a while, then put the phone away. After a short while, sometimes just two or three minutes, they repeat the process. And they do this time and again.

Anybody would agree that these are signs of a serious addiction. How can you avoid this? If already caught up in the process, how can you eliminate that behavior?

Solution

The urge to pick up an electronic device and use it comes from the subconscious. How can we counteract that unbidden demand?

A story about my friend Manfried[116] provides a clue. We had arrived at a small airport in Montana for a week of camping and hiking, and I had gone to pick up the rental car.

Getting the car turned out to be a drawn-out process, and I returned to Manfried after more than 45 minutes. My apology "Sorry it took so long. You must have been really bored" drew from Manfried the surprising response "Don't worry. I am never bored."

Curious, I asked, "How come you are never bored?" He answered, "There is always something interesting to watch."

Manfried's wonderful insight can be the basis for a mantra. Whenever the unbidden thought "This is really boring" surfaces and we are tempted to open up an electronic device for entertainment, we invoke the counteracting mantra "Let's observe what's going on."

Will this suffice to overcome the addiction to profit media? It's enough for Manfried, who uses his innate gift to marvel at the world. For most everybody else, the mantra will fail to stop the addiction.

But the story has at its core a key insight: If we are to conquer the addiction, we must engage in some interesting and satisfying activity that replaces the mind-numbing interaction with electronics.

The replacement comes in various versions. For example, we may engage in a physical activity where we create something with our hands, we talk with a friend, or we may get together with people important to us. There is a common thread to the diversity: For a hunter-gatherer, each of these activities was important for survival. Why is that so?

Evolution changed humans so that activities fostering survival became desirable and produced feelings of accomplishment and pleasure. Put differently, evolution created subconscious neuroprocesses that produce deep satisfaction whenever we carry out these activities. We can enhance the effectiveness using modern technology. For example, instead of meeting with a friend, we call them on the phone or via Skype.

In contrast, the electronic blips of digital media interchanges may feel good for a fleeting moment, but have no lasting impact. That's because evolution didn't create any subconscious neuroprocesses that convert momentary blips of information into feelings of accomplishment.

The book *Digital Minimalism: Choosing a Focused Life in a Noisy World*[117] by C. Newport works out this observation in detail and suggests the following: As a first step, we should create a number of activities where we interact with the world. The exact form is not important. What counts is that the activities produce great satisfaction.

We can test if an activity qualifies. That is, we strip away the technology and identify the essential process. It is guaranteed to be important if the simplified activity was important for the survival of hunter-gatherers.

For example, creating and building things was important, as was communication with friends, for example, for effective hunting. The same applied to meeting with members of the clan to assure mutual support in difficult endeavors.

Once we have installed the new activities, we begin to eliminate profit media interaction.

That process has an important component: Each time an unbidden thought surfaces to interact with media, you tell yourself, "This isn't good for me. Let's do something else, maybe just watch what's going on around me."

That mantra slowly changes subconscious neuroprocesses to the point where any temptation offered by media triggers a thought of irritation if not disgust such as "Just forget this stuff."

Interestingly enough, the same method works when we fight *any* addiction, as described in *Dopamine Nation: Finding Balance in the Age of Indulgence*[118] by A. Lembke. That is, we first identify alternate, satisfying behavior, then we devise schemes that eliminate addictive actions.

Getting Started

We begin the withdrawal process with a drastic step and simply shut down interaction with profit media for several weeks. The recommended period is four weeks.

That number agrees with a general recommendation for the fight against any addiction, as described in *Dopamine Nation*: Completely avoid any and all actions of the addiction for four weeks.

Generally speaking, the first two weeks of that period entail serious withdrawal symptoms. They lessen during the subsequent two weeks. At the end of that time, the urge of the addiction typically has subsided.

We finish our discussion about profit media, its devious actions, and how we can escape them. If you want to learn more about profit media, the withdrawal process, and subsequent reduced if not eliminated use, go to the books *Digital Minimalism* and *Dopamine Nation*.

Seemingly independent of, but actually connected with, the fight against any addiction is the proposal of the next chapter: Every day we should reserve a period where we rest our mind.

23

Meditation

How come Manfried of Chapter 22 can always identify some interesting things or activities in the world and thus never gets bored? The answer: He has a natural gift for observing the world.

Not everyone is so lucky. In fact, our interaction with the world via models, as described in Chapter 4, pushes us to *not* observe details of the world and instead rely on stored models. The efficiency with which we sometimes make decisions in a fraction of a second relies on that preference.

How, then, can we make observation of the world interesting? We somehow must turn off the models at times, become childlike in our curiosity, and thus become directly connected with the world and its multitude of events and processes.

Restoring Curiosity

One tool can restore childlike attention to the world: Meditation.

You may pause for a moment and look up the "Meditation" entry of the Wikipedia. It's an amazing assembly of diverse human thought on various ways to change our lives.

We shall not attempt even a cursory overview of the possibilities. Instead, we focus on one particular approach that is easy to learn and doesn't require much time every day. It not only relaxes us and strips away the tension of the day, but also sharpens our attention so that we can focus on details of the world.

The technique is *mindfulness*.[119]

It creates a value system that rejects proposals such as "Work hard and play harder," and instead allows us to experience the world in all its richness without the artificial machinery of electronics.

Mindfulness

An important part of mindfulness is a *body-scan technique* where we lie down, relax, let breathing and pulse stabilize, and gradually survey the body. We experience what each body part feels at the moment. The effect is that we not only learn to listen to our body, but also become sensitive to the world around us.

The body-scan technique requires determined training[120] in which we follow the steps of the program every day.

In the language of subconscious models, we gradually install a new way of viewing the world.

At the end of each session we congratulate ourselves for having done the meditation and end with a strong, positive feeling.

After a few days, we begin to feel more connected with the world. When we take a walk in the park, admiring the beauty of trees and lakes and birds, we look at other walkers staring at a phone with mild amazement. Why don't they see the beauty around them instead of focusing on a tiny glass plate with miniature pictures and text?

Later, we learn to enjoy the meditation process itself: It is a nice experience, independent of the fact that it produces a richer and more relaxed life.

Later still, we realize that our entire lives can be viewed as a meditative process. At that point, we have become a different person.

All this means: We never become bored. Our friend Manfried achieved this naturally, without any particular effort. We can get there through meditation.

The effect of the meditation isn't just that we look at the world differently. Here are three examples.

Relaxation

Due to meditation we often move into a state of relaxation without conscious effort. Say, we are participating in a tense meeting at the office. As we sit there and listen to heated arguments, we suddenly feel our body becoming relaxed. Mentally we are stepping back from the scene. At the same time we sense how irrelevant that discussion really is, and that we should just sit and listen.

Anger Management

Mindfulness meditation prepares us well for anger management.

During a meeting at the office, somebody launches a heated attack on us. At first we feel annoyed, and then angry.

What should we do? In childhood we learned to fight back, using our anger as a driving force. If we do so, our anger will rise as we respond. Then there will be counterarguments and even angrier reactions by us.

Not good, is it?

Buddhism has an alternate approach.[121] It views our rising anger as both a problem and an opportunity where we learn and grow. That is, the attacking opponent is not a foe, but makes it possible for us to practice effective anger management.

How can we achieve this? We invoke the thought "I feel the rising anger. Let's use this opportunity to practice anger management and to learn and grow." That thought disconnects the anger from us and turns it into an opportunity, an amazing transformation.

We can learn this reaction by thinking daily about it and invoking the above statement as a mantra. The subconscious then produces that thought whenever we feel a rising anger.

When we have handled a case of anger this way, with us calm and relaxed throughout, we tell ourselves, "Hey, isn't it great how we handled this situation and became better at handling anger?"

Mindfulness training helps us slow down our response when somebody's anger assaults us, and thus gives us time to invoke the mantra and start the correct reaction.

Escape From Profit Media

Meditation is another tool in the fight of addiction to profit media. That is, meditation teaches us to recognize and respond to the richness of the world, and thus lets us see the electronic blip communication of profit media as fleeting and largely irrelevant.

We stop here with the second part and begin the third part. It concerns Life. "Oh my," you are likely to think, "how can anybody say anything meaningful about that complex topic in a few chapters?"

Let's try.

Part III

Life

24

Getting Old

It's New Year's Eve. You promise your partner that you resolve to exercise more. The next four weeks you do so, but then old habits resurface. Exercise is a fad, isn't it? It doesn't matter what you do, eventually you will die anyway, won't you? A friend tells you, "The people who exercise don't get to be older. They just *look* older." You agree and find this funny.

You are past 50. On vacation in the mountains, you talk with people much younger than you. They hike long, steep trails up to mountain peaks. You know that at your age that is no longer possible. You nod wistfully as they describe their day since you used to take such hikes. Instead, you take a Jeep tour to experience the views. You are just too old for strenuous hikes, aren't you?

You are approaching 60. Walking up the staircase to the second floor of the office building becomes difficult. You are running out of breath and are panting when you reach the top. You decide that walking the staircase is no longer good for you and take the elevator. That's why there are elevators, aren't there?

You are at the official retirement age, 67. There is a short ceremony at the office. Your colleagues tell you that you will be missed, and congratulate you that you finally will be able to relax. You go home and relax indeed: You get up late in the morning, dawdle throughout the day, and in the evening watch TV. A life of true leisure.

When somebody asks you about your retirement, you say, "It's great." You no longer work hard. After all, wear and tear causes illness and death, doesn't it? But deep down you sense a difficult-to-describe loss.

Is there a common thread connecting these depressing conclusions?

Shortcomings of Evolution

Chapter 12 provides a clue: It shows that evolution did not install the correct reaction to a hurt shoulder or lower back. Indeed, evolution didn't have to since the daily activities required for survival of hunter-gatherers were the correct response.

Identical arguments apply to the above, dismal conclusions: Hunter-gatherers were physically active every day, they had no time for vacation, there were no helpful elevators, and retirement was an unknown concept.

Hence evolution never had to handle the problems of aging. In the terminology used in this book, the subconscious and conscious neuroprocesses shaped by evolution are not designed to cope with these difficulties.

"Wait a moment," you might say, "this hunter-gatherer argument doesn't apply. Their life expectancy was somewhere between 20 and 35 years, and getting old never was a problem." While the cited average lifespan is correct, the argument overlooks that 70% of deaths were due to disease and 20% were caused by violence or accidents. Those not afflicted by those factors lived well into their 60s and even early 70s.[122]

How can we overcome the problem that evolution hasn't prepared us for the aging process? Corrective actions for the previous cases provide a clue, as we see next.

25

Staying Young

Two events bracket our life: birth and death. Nobody asked us whether we wanted to be born, and death will happen eventually no matter what. So let's ignore what we can't do anything about, and instead focus on the in-between time: our life.

We get some idea how we should conduct our life by solving the problems raised in Chapters 12.

Suppose we have hurt ourselves by falling or tripping. The ensuing pain is supposed to reduce activities so that the body can repair the damage. We have seen that this can be quite the wrong reaction.

We avoid this by consulting well-established websites[123] for advice. In the specific case of the hurt shoulder, we should gently exercise movement of the shoulder. That way the shoulder heals while retaining its flexibility. For the problem of a hurt back, a number of yoga exercises promote healing and strengthening of the back.

In severe cases, the family doctor will prescribe rehab treatment by a specialist. Regardless of the case, we do not follow the gut reaction that healing can only take place when we don't exercise the hurting part of our body.

Let's turn to the gradual deterioration of abilities from age 50 onward. It is widely accepted as part of aging. Why fight what nature will force anyway? This is a self-fulfilling prophecy. By doing less and less, we become less and less capable. It's triggered by the fact that evolution didn't design subconscious and conscious neuroprocesses for decisions to scale back, for the simple reason that hunter-gatherers never had that option.

What should we do then? Bluntly speaking, we override the bad decisions with better choices, as follows.

The Plan

While we are still in good shape, we introduce exercises that determine what we can do. If we discover that our capabilities are too limited, we work to expand the horizon of activities.

For example, if we aren't able to bend forward and touch the ground with our fingertips without flexing the knees, we exercise to gradually achieve this. After a while, we not only can do this, but may even be able to place our hands flat on the ground.

The same goes for everything else: We establish that we can walk certain distances, climb stairs with reasonable speed, hike in the mountains, swim certain distances. We don't need to do *all* of this, but do *much* of it. In some sense, we establish a reasonable level of overall physical capacity.

Daily we carry out a program of exercises to maintain that level. The program can be broken up into parts if you prefer that. We also may declare one day of each week to be a holiday from the exercises, say Saturday or Sunday.

Now and then we notice that something isn't working anymore as it should. We develop a back pain, say. We inquire how this can be fixed by additional exercise, and add that new activity to the program.

You say, "Whoa, does this mean that the program is gradually expanding?" Indeed, that is the message.

It is the exact opposite of what common wisdom decrees, where our body gradually becomes less and less capable and we correspond by doing less and less.

Satisfaction

As the years roll by, your daily maintenance activities expand. Each day you complete them, you congratulate yourself for having done so. Lo and behold, you begin to look forward to them as a nice part of your day.

An amazing result? Not really. Cognitive behavioral therapy (CBT) predicts that this will happen.

Benefits

Your program produces two key results.

First, you stay fit to continue all the activities you love to do. Riding a bike, hiking in the mountains, swimming in the ocean, flying an airplane, building furniture, repairing the house, maintaining your car, and so on. Whatever it is, you can continue doing it.

Second, your nervous system remains in excellent condition for the intellectual endeavors you like to pursue:[124] Reading books of fiction as well as nonfiction, for example, about advances in the natural and social sciences, mathematics, and the arts; attending lectures at the local community college or university and learning innumerable interesting facts; acquiring a new language; sketching or painting indoors and outdoors; writing a blog about particular aspects of life and the world; and so on.

In short, you have a rich and satisfying life.

Retirement

"Wait a minute!" you say, "How about retirement and a relaxed life?" Forget retirement and a relaxed life. That is, you may quit your regular job at any age once you have become financially independent using the strategy of Chapter 19. But then you pick up something else that you carry out with equal commitment.

When somebody asks you, "When are you going to retire?" you respond with the following.

> "Let me describe the day I retire. In the morning I won't feel well. At noon I will go to the hospital, and at nightfall I will be dead."

———————————

There is more to consider, as we see in the next chapter.

26

Ikigai

The Japanese word "ikigai" (pronounced ick-ee-guy) translates directly to "life's purpose." Other versions are "a reason for living," "a meaning of life," and "what makes life worth living."[125]

The statements refer to an extensive philosophy of life practiced in Japan that according to one study decreases the risk of mortality.[126]

What does ikigai entail? When you investigate this question, you come upon a variety of claims.[127]

Here are ten recommendations taken from *Ikigai: The Japanese Secret To a Long and Happy Life*[128] by H. Garcia and F. Miralles. We include a comment with each case.

- *Stay active; don't retire.* Chapter 25 has details.
- *Take it slow.* Step away from the hustle and bustle. Meditation teaches you how to do this; see Chapter 23.
- *Don't fill your stomach.* Chapter 9 warns of the perils of overeating and how to avoid them. Ikigai recommends eating to 80% full.
- *Surround yourself with good friends.* It's interesting that ikigai points out the importance of human connection. Evolution has created the subconscious drive to stay connected with others. Modern life makes these connections more difficult, so we need to consciously establish them.
- *Get in shape.* Chapter 25 shows that exercise is hugely important.

- *Smile.* What an interesting concept! Very useful, too. Friendly interactions with family, friends, casual acquaintances, even strangers add a pleasant glow to life.

- *Reconnect with nature.* Another important point. Technology tends to put up barriers between us and nature, and we must deliberately act to reconnect. Examples are hiking in the mountains, swimming in the ocean, visiting botanical gardens and zoos, and creating our own small world of nature in the backyard.

- *Give thanks.* Often overlooked, but so important. By thanking we connect with others in a fundamental way. We can also give thanks for our fortunate circumstances by helping others, see Chapter 19.

- *Live in the moment.* Chapter 23 describes how meditation restores our curiosity about the world and thus connects us more closely with our environment.

- *Follow your ikigai.* Discover what your passion is and let it drive you.

Beyond This Book

It's easy to see that ikigai doesn't cover all important considerations for life; for example, how we should handle pain, cope with digital media, or counter the onslaught of drugs.

But then this book isn't complete, either, and one can always say more about life and errant subconscious neuroprocesses.

It's an unavoidable shortcoming. But having worked through the cases of this book, you are well equipped to recognize and deal with subconscious blunders as they come up.

Part IV

Epilogue

Our prior book *Magic, Error, and Terror*[129] explored how subconscious and conscious models may help, trouble, or harm us in a number of settings.

The subsequent book *Wittgenstein and Brain Science*[130] showed that a number of philosophical problems haven't been solved due to a fundamental erroneous assumption about human reasoning that ignores the complex functioning of the nervous system.

The most recent book *Artificial Intelligence*[131] used results of neuroscience to establish why research projects in AI fail or succeed. In particular, the book illuminates why AI research of the first 40 years failed completely, and why we still have failures mixed in with the rather recent successes.

This book is our fourth investigation how the results of modern neuroscience impact our understanding of the world. It focuses on the unreliability of the subconscious neuroprocesses when their output directly affects our well-being.

To be sure, mistakes of the subconscious neuroprocesses have always existed and thus have created trouble for mankind. It's part of being human.

But in recent decades, industry has exploited shortcomings of the subconscious neuroprocesses on a truly terrifying scale. That's on top of the awful impact of the modern sedentary lifestyle.

We, the victims of that development, can fight against the disastrous outcomes by identifying the root causes and then adopting corrective actions. This includes changes of flawed subconscious neuroprocesses through conscious thoughts, as proposed by cognitive behavioral therapy (CBT).

A Personal Note

I have implemented everything described here. Some changes required some effort while others were easily accomplished. For example, development of an appropriate physical exercise program took some time, while control of the profit media was simple since I never suffered from the serious addiction described in *Digital Minimalism*.[132]

My personal experience confirms the positive results achieved by others, as covered in Parts I–III.

Indeed, through appropriate choices and changes, *everyone* can do much better, stay much healthier, remain amazingly active, and overall experience a richer life.

Notes

The notes frequently refer to Wikipedia since it is readily accessible without charge. Unless otherwise indicated, it is the English version.
The Wikipedia entries often supply an extensive list of references for additional explanations. Pointing to the entry spares us from listing all those references.
Better yet, as insight into a topic grows, Wikipedia changes as well. Hence the reader always obtains the latest information about the topic.
All links were verified in fall 2023.

Chapter 1 Introduction

1. In this chapter, the term "conscious mind" refers to the part of the brain whose performance we are aware of. Chapter 15 expands that definition to include the awareness itself.

2. In 2023, Twitter was renamed to "X." We always use the original name since it is well-known while "X" may cause confusion depending on context.

3. [Fisher, 2022].

4. See Wikipedia "Rohingya genocide."

5. [Moss, 2013].

6. See Wikipedia "Obesity in the United States" for detailed historical statistics on obesity. The Center for Disease Control and Prevention (CDC) supplied the obesity statistic for 2022. See https://www.cdc.gov/obesity/data/adult.html.

7. See Wikipedia "Opioid epidemic in the United States."

8. See Wikipedia "Problematic social media use," "Digital media use and mental health," and "Social media and suicide."

9. At present, social media, the food processing industry, and the pharmaceutical companies exert enormous influence over the political processes. The lobbying efforts are so strong and effective that politicians are unable to implement even modest changes. Only time will tell if that destructive effort can be stopped.

10. [Kahneman, 2011].

11. [Chabris and Simons, 2011].

12. [Myers, 2002].

13. In 2023, a search of the Amazon website using the key word "overthinking" produced more than 30 titles.

14. [Trenton, 2021].

15. [Shell, 2003].

16. [Moss, 2013].

17. [Newport, 2019].

18. [Fisher, 2022].

19. [Lembke, 2021].

Chapter 2 Nervous System

20. [Truemper, 2021].

21. [Truemper, 2023].

22. See Wikipedia "Outline of the human nervous system."

23. Source: "Nervous system diagram." By Medium69, Jmarchn, CC BY-SA 4.0 https://commons.wikimedia.org/wiki/File:Nervous_system_diagram-en.svg, via Wikimedia Commons.

Chapter 3 Cold and Hot

24. An example of a potentially dangerous situation is swimming

in hot water, say of 92 deg F. If we swim slowly, this will not cause a problem. But when done with substantial effort, the body will heat up and will try to fight the rising temperature with profuse sweating. However, the sweat is absorbed by the water, and there is no cooling effect. The sweating rapidly dehydrates the body, causing muscle spasms and possibly life-threatening arrhythmia. See https://www.drweil.com/health-wellness/health-centers/children/too-hot-to-swim/.

Chapter 4 Models

25. The postulate is consistent with the neuroscience theory of predictive coding, also called predictive processing. The theory says that the brain constantly generates and updates a so-called mental model of the environment; see Wikipedia "Predictive coding." The postulate introduced here is consistent with the theory of predictive coding, but goes further since it claims a universal role of models for the entire nervous system.

26. [Hawking and Mlodinow, 2010]. The concept of model-dependent realism is more elaborate than Plato's much-cited claim "Reality is created by the mind. We can change reality by changing our mind" https://wiseowlquotes.com/plato/. Indeed, Plato doesn't differentiate between conscious and subconscious models, nor does he consider the complex ways in which subconscious models can be changed by conscious thoughts, as discussed in Chapter 6.

Chapter 5 Creation of Models

27. [Truemper, 2021] discusses model errors in various settings.

Chapter 6 Remedy

28. [Burns, 2020] provides not only a clear introduction, but is sufficiently detailed for readers who are looking for solutions they can implement by themselves.

29. See Wikipedia "Cognitive behavioral therapy." For treatment examples, see [Beck et al., 1979], [Burns, 2008], and [Burns, 2020]. [Truemper, 2021] describes a composite case.

30. See Wikipedia "Heart rate."

31. The advice is based on the title of [Carlson, 1997].

Chapter 7 Food and Drink

32. The technical term is "oral cavity." It includes the lips, the lining inside the cheeks and lips, the front two thirds of the tongue, the upper and lower gums, the floor of the mouth under the tongue, the bony roof of the mouth, and the small area behind the wisdom teeth. See https://www.cancer.gov/publications/dictionaries/cancer-terms/def/oral-cavity.

33. See Wikipedia "Enteric nervous system." We are tempted to propose that the parts of the nervous system that evaluate food in the mouth be considered part of the ENS. For example, if totally disgusting food is detected in the mouth, it may cause the stomach to heave.

34. See Wikipedia "Enteric nervous system."

Chapter 8 Sugar, Fat, and Salt

35. For simplicity of discussion, we use the term "sugar" to refer to sugar and any one of its substitutes such as high-fructose corn syrup.

36. [Moss, 2013].

37. See Wikipedia "Ultra-processed food."

Chapter 9 A Health Crisis

38. Chapter 2 [Shell, 2003].

39. See Wikipedia "Obesity in the United States" for detailed historical statistics on obesity. The Center for Disease Control and Prevention (CDC) supplied the obesity statistics for 2022. See https://www.cdc.gov/obesity/data/adult.html.

40. [Gupta et al., 2019].

41. See Wikipedia "Obesity." The impact of obesity on anxiety, depression, and cognitive decline is only partially understood; see New York Times "The Link Between Highly Processed Foods and Brain Health" by Sally Wadyka, May 4, 2023; https://www.nytime

s.com/2023/05/04/well/eat/ultraprocessed-food-mental-healt
h.html.

42. Complete instructions about baking bread, rolls, and baguettes with sourdough are available at https://afewcreativesolutions.com/2018/07/23/baking-sourdough-rye-bread-overview/#more-253.

43. See Wikipedia "Mediterranean diet."

44. See Wikipedia "DASH diet."

45. See Wikipedia "MIND diet."

46. [Greger, 2015].

47. [Moss, 2013].

48. Sourdough bread photos: copyright 2018 K. Truemper. Released into Public Domain under Creative Commons CC0. Details about baking bread, rolls, and baguettes with sourdough are available at https://afewcreativesolutions.com/2018/07/23/baking-sourdough-rye-bread-overview/#more-253.

Chapter 10 Breathless

49. This chapter is adopted from the book *Magic, Error, and Terror* [Truemper, 2021]. The first part is based on Wikipedia "Chronic obstructive pulmonary disease."

50. [Nestor, 2020].

51. See Wikipedia "Medulla oblongata."

52. Source: "Medulla of brain" by OpenStax - https://cnx.org/contents/FPtK1zmh@8.25:fEI3C80t@10/Preface, CC BY 4.0, https://commons.wikimedia.org/w/index.php?curid=30147954.

53. The discussion is based on [Nestor, 2020].

54. p. 76 [Nestor, 2020].

55. The extreme case is hyperventilation, where more CO_2 is eliminated by the lungs than produced by the body. See Wikipedia "Hyperventilation."

56. p. 81 [Nestor, 2020].

57. See Wikipedia "Panic attack." Chapter 3 [Truemper, 2021] discusses the treatment of panic attacks in the framework of conscious and subconscious neuroprocesses.

58. [Nestor, 2020].

Chapter 11 Fatigue

59. Chapter 4 [Truemper, 2021] supplies part of the material of this chapter.

60. Craig Glenday, Editor-in-Chief at Guinness World Records, reported:
"Georges Holtyzer of Belgium walked 673.48 km (418.49 miles) in 6 days 10 hr 58 min, completing 452 laps of a 1.49 km (0.92 mile) circuit at Ninove, Belgium, from July 19 to July 25, 1986. He was not permitted any stops for rest and was moving 98.78 percent of the time."
The quote was available on the Internet in 2021, but by 2023 was replaced by a shorter statement available at https://www.quora.com/ What-is-the-longest-distance-a-person-has-walked-in-one-go.

61. p. 209 [Grafton, 2020].

62. p. 210, 211 [Grafton, 2020].

63. p. 213 [Grafton, 2020].

64. See Wikipedia "Paavo Nurmi."

65. p. 214 [Grafton, 2020].

66. [Gibson et al., 2013] describes three stages of collapse.

- During the early stage—the "Early Foster" collapse position—the runner exhibits unstable gait and lowers the head.
- The gait deteriorates to a shuffle in the "Half Foster" collapse position, with head parallel to the ground.
- In the final stage—the "Full Foster" collapse position—the runner crawls on the ground on elbows and knees and finally collapses before or after reaching the finish line.

The reference conjectures that the collapse positions are indicative of a final, likely primordial, protective mechanism.

67. We have been unable to trace the origin of the grape process. Two pilots told us about it and assured us it works every time.

68. See the post `https://pointsforpilots.blogspot.com/2023/05/fatigue-in-cockpit.html`.

69. Chapter 3 [Truemper, 2021] describes how subconscious models produce panic attacks, and how cognitive behavioral therapy (CBT) can change these models.

Chapter 12 Pain

70. See Wikipedia "Low back pain."

71. See the video `https://en.wikipedia.org/wiki/File:Low_Back_Pain.webm`.

72. [Lembke, 2021] discusses the operation of the balance scale in great detail.

73. [Lembke, 2021].

Chapter 13 A Flood of Drugs

74. The discussion about drugs and their abuse applies to the US. Quite different situations exist elsewhere. For example, the pricing and use of drugs in Western Europe is tightly regulated.

75. See Wikipedia "Fentanyl."

76. See Wikipedia "Osteoporosis."

77. See the Better Health Channel of the Department of Health, Victoria State, Australia, `https://www.betterhealth.vic.gov.au/health/conditionsandtreatments/osteoporosis`.

78. See Wikipedia "Spaceflight osteopenia."

79. See Wikipedia "Dual-energy X-ray absorptiometry."

80. See Wikipedia "Fosamax."

81. See Wikipedia "Obesity in the United States" for detailed historical statistics on obesity. The Center for Disease Control and Prevention (CDC) supplied the obesity statistics for 2022. See `https://www.cdc.gov/obesity/data/adult.html`.

82. See Wikipedia "Anti-obesity medication" for the extensive list of drugs combatting obesity.

83. See https://www.medicalnewstoday.com/articles/drugs-wego vy-side-effects.

84. If Medicare covers the new brand-name obesity drugs, they could cost $13 to $26 billion dollars per year even with only 10% of people with obesity using them. See https://www.vumc.org/healt h-policy/medicare-antiobesity-medications-nejm.

Chapter 14 Alternatives

85. For several decades, Joe and Terry Graedon have been teaching, writing, and broadcasting information about health problems and their resolution. The People's Pharmacy website https://www.peop lespharmacy.com/about is the gateway to that information.

86. [Greger, 2015].

87. A low-cost source of goldenrod is Mountain Rose Herbs https://mountainroseherbs.com/goldenrod.

Chapter 15 Mind Definition

88. See Wikipedia "Mind."

89. p. 3 [Truemper, 2022].

Chapter 16 A Dead-Sure Investor

90. It is ironic that in 2022 the stock price of the company was at its highest value ever and 7.5 times the price when John sold his entire holdings.

Chapter 17 Bad Advice

91. See, for example, "How to Invest in Stocks: A Beginner's Guide for Getting Started," https://www.fool.com/investing/how-to-in vest/stocks/.

92. The comparison with a fox guarding the hen house is not overly harsh. The famous investment book *The Four Pillars of Investing* by W. Bernstein [Bernstein, 2023] has the following, even stronger statement:
"...you won't go far wrong by treating the entire financial services

industry as a battlefield—certainly any stockbroker or full-service brokerage firm, any newsletter, any advisor who purchases individual securities, and any hedge fund. It's not too much of an exaggeration to say that the average stockbroker services his clients in the same way that [the infamous American bank robber] Baby Face Nelson serviced banks."

Chapter 18 Mistakes

93. See Worldodometer https://www.worldometers.info/computers/ for the total number of computers and the number sold during the current year.

94. See Wikipedia "Ponzi scheme."

95. See Wikipedia "Subprime mortgage crisis."

Chapter 19 Solution

96. See Wikipedia "John C. Bogle."

97. See Wikipedia "John C. Bogle."

98. S&P Dow Jones Indices LLC produces, maintains, licenses, and markets the S&P 500 index as well as other market indices. See Wikipedia "S&P Dow Jones Indices."

99. See Wikipedia "Vanguard index funds."

100. Vanguard states these facts as follows on their website https://investor.vanguard.com/corporate-portal/:
"Vanguard isn't owned by shareholders. It's owned by the people who invest in our funds.
"As an owner you have access to personalized financial advice, high-quality investments, retirement tools, and relevant market insights ... "

101. The fact that any small successful company either will be bought by a company in the S&P 500 index or will enter the index by itself, illuminates why another index that covers the entire stock market—the Total Stock Market index—behaves essentially the same way as the S&P 500 index:
The S&P 500 index reflects the performance of large and generally successful companies plus that of successful companies acquired by them. The Total Stock Market index is the S&P 500 index ad-

justed by the performance of all small companies, some successful and not yet acquired by large companies, and the rest unsuccessful. The net effect of that adjustment turns out to be insignificant.

Chapter 20 Digital Media

102. [Fisher, 2022].

103. [Fisher, 2022].

104. See Wikipedia "Rohingya genocide."

105. See Wikipedia "Problematic social media use," "Digital media use and mental health," and "Social media and suicide."

106. [Newport, 2019].

107. [Lembke, 2021].

Chapter 21 Economics and Evolution

108. https://www.wikipedia.org/.

109. https://archive.org/.

110. https://www.nytimes.com/.

111. https://www.facebook.com/.

112. https://twitter.com/X.

113. https://www.google.com.

114. https://www.bing.com/.

115. p. 8, 9 [Newport, 2019], emphasis in original.

Chapter 22 Escape From Profit Media

116. Manfried is the actual name. He was a friend for 60 years.

117. [Newport, 2019].

118. [Lembke, 2021].

Chapter 23 Meditation

119. For a number of books on mindfulness, including the classic [Kabat-Zinn, 1990], see Wikipedia "Jon Kabat-Zinn."

120. Various mindfulness training programs can be downloaded free of charge: http://www.freemindfulness.org/download. In the discussion of this chapter, we specifically mean the program "Forty five minute body scan." It requires 45 minutes, as stated in the title. But later, when you have become good at the body scan, you can reduce it to something like 20 minutes, done each day.

121. The 14th Dalai Lama has done much to bring these thoughts to the Western World. Search the Internet for "books by the Dalai Lama." The arguments cited here are taken from [His Holiness The Dalai Lama and Cutler, 2009].

Chapter 24 Getting Old

122. See Wikipedia "Hunter-gatherer" and Encyclopedia of Evolutionary Psychological Science "Life Expectancy in Hunter-Gatherers."

Chapter 25 Staying Young

123. Reliable sources are, for example, the Mayo Clinic https://www.mayoclinic.org/ and the National Institute of Health (NIH) https://www.nih.gov/.

124. Extensive literature covers the benefits of physical activity on cognitive control; see summary in [Skolasinska et al., 2023]. The reference supplies important results how strenuous physical activity and cardiorespiratory fitness avoid age-related neurocognitive decline.

Chapter 26 Ikigai

125. See Wikipedia "*Ikigai.*"

126. [Tanno et al., 2009].

127. The Internet supplies several definitions and viewpoints about ikigai. For example, https://modelthinkers.com/mental-model/ikigai lists the following four rules: Do

- What you love
- What you are good at
- What the world needs
- What you can be paid for

In contrast, [Mogi, 2018] claims the following five pillars:

- Starting small → Focusing on the details.
- Releasing yourself → Accepting who you are.
- Harmony and sustainability → Relying on others.
- The joy of little things → Appreciating sensory pleasure.
- Being in the here and now → Finding your flow.

Confusing, isn't it? The lack of clarity stems from the fact that there is no a priori definition of ikigai. Instead, some people observed Japanese men and women who claim to live according to ikigai, then deduced rules and principles from that information. This also applies to the ten recommendations cited in the text.

The lack of a clear definition is reflected in the sometimes heated discussion about ikigai in the Wikipedia Talk section of *"Ikigai"*; see `https://en.wikipedia.org/wiki/Talk:Ikigai`.

128. [Garcis and Miralles, 2017].

Epilogue

129. [Truemper, 2021].

130. [Truemper, 2022].

131. [Truemper, 2023].

132. [Newport, 2019].

Bibliography

[Beck et al., 1979] Beck, A. T., Rush, A. J., Shaw, B. F., and Emery, G. (1979). *Cognitive Therapy of Depression*. Guilford Press.

[Bernstein, 2023] Bernstein, W. (2023). *The Four Pillars of Investing: Lessons for Building a Winning Portfolio*. McGraw Hill, second edition.

[Burns, 2008] Burns, D. D. (2008). *Feeling Good: The New Mood Therapy*. Harper.

[Burns, 2020] Burns, D. D. (2020). *Feeling Great: The Revolutionary New Treatment for Depression and Anxiety*. PESI Publishing & Media.

[Carlson, 1997] Carlson, R. (1997). *Don't Sweat the Small Stuff . . . It's All Small Stuff: Simple Ways to Keep the Little Things from Taking Over Your Life*. Hachette Books.

[Chabris and Simons, 2011] Chabris, C. and Simons, D. (2011). *The Invisible Gorilla: How Our Intuitions Deceive Us*. Broadway Paperbacks.

[Fisher, 2022] Fisher, M. (2022). *The Chaos Machine: The Inside Story of How Social Media Rewired Our Minds and Our World*. Hachette Book Group, Inc.

[Garcis and Miralles, 2017] Garcis, H. and Miralles, F. (2017). *Ikigai: The Japanese Secret to a Long and Happy Life*. Penguin Books.

[Gibson et al., 2013] Gibson, A. S. C., De Koning, J. J., Thompson, K. G., Roberts, W. O., Micklewright, D., Raglin, J., and Foster, C.

(2013). Crawling to the finish line: why do endurance runners collapse? Implications for understanding of mechanisms underlying pacing and fatigue. *Sports Medicine*, vol. 43, pp. 413–424.

[Grafton, 2020] Grafton, S. (2020). *Physical Intelligence: The Science of How the Body and the Mind Guide Each Other Through Life*. Penguin Random House.

[Greger, 2015] Greger, M. (2015). *How Not to Die: Discover the Foods Scientifically Proven to Prevent and Reverse Disease*. Flatiron Books.

[Gupta et al., 2019] Gupta, S., Hawk, T., Aggarwal, A., and Drewnowski, A. (2019). Characterizing Ultra-Processed Foods by Energy Density, Nutrient Density, and Cost. *Frontiers of Nutrition*, May 28, 2019. https://pubmed.ncbi.nlm.nih.gov/3123 1655/.

[Hawking and Mlodinow, 2010] Hawking, S. and Mlodinow, L. (2010). *The Grand Design*. Bantam Books.

[His Holiness The Dalai Lama and Cutler, 2009] His Holiness The Dalai Lama and Cutler, H. C. (2009). *The Art of Happiness*. Riverhead Books.

[Kabat-Zinn, 1990] Kabat-Zinn, J. (1990). *Full Catastrophe Living*. Dell Publishing.

[Kahneman, 2011] Kahneman, D. (2011). *Thinking, Fast and Slow*. Farrar, Straus, and Giroux.

[Lembke, 2021] Lembke, A. (2021). *Dopamine Nation: Finding Balance in the Age of Indulgence*. Dutton.

[Mogi, 2018] Mogi, K. (2018). *Awakening Your Ikigai: How the Japanese Wake Up to Joy and Purpose Every Day*. The Experiment.

[Moss, 2013] Moss, M. (2013). *Salt Sugar Fat: How the Food Giants Hooked Us*. Random House.

[Myers, 2002] Myers, D. G. (2002). *Intuition: Its Powers and Perils*. Yale University Press.

[Nestor, 2020] Nestor, J. (2020). *Breath: The New Science of a Lost Art*. Riverhead Books.

[Newport, 2019] Newport, C. (2019). *Digital Minimalism: Choosing a Focused Life in a Noisy World*. Penguin Random House.

[Shell, 2003] Shell, E. R. (2003). *The Hungry Gene: The Inside Story of the Obesity Crisis*. Grove Press.

[Skolasinska et al., 2023] Skolasinska, P., Basak, C., and Qin, S. (2023). Influence of strenuous physical activity and cardiorespiratory fitness on age-related differences in brain activations during varieties of cognitive control. *Neuroscience*, vol. 520, pp. 58-83.

[Tanno et al., 2009] Tanno, K., Sakata, K., Ohsawa, M., Onoda, T., Itai, K., Yaegashi, Y., and Tamakoshi, A. (2009). Associations of ikigai as a positive psychological factor with all-cause mortality and cause-specific mortality among middle-aged and elderly Japanese people: Findings from the Japan Collaborative Cohort Study. *J. of Psychosomatic Research*, vol. 67, pp. 67-75.

[Trenton, 2021] Trenton, N. (2021). *Stop Overthinking: 23 Techniques to Relieve Stress, Stop Negative Spirals, Declutter Your Mind, and Focus on the Present*. independently published.

[Truemper, 2021] Truemper, K. (2021). *Magic, Error, and Terror: How Models in Our Brain Succeed and Fail*. Leibniz Company.

[Truemper, 2022] Truemper, K. (2022). *Wittgenstein and Brain Science: Understanding the World*. Leibniz Company.

[Truemper, 2023] Truemper, K. (2023). *Artificial Intelligence: Why AI Projects Succeed or Fail*. Leibniz Company.

Acknowledgements

Technical advice, evaluation of chapters, corrections, or general help were provided by C. Basak, M. Grötschel, M. Opperud, and M. Steigleder.

I. Truemper and U. Truemper were patient editors.

The University of Texas at Dallas—our home institution—made essential resources available.

We thank all of them for their help.

K. T.

Index

www.ingramcontent.com/pod-product-compliance
Lightning Source LLC
Chambersburg PA
CBHW032002040426
42448CB00006B/454